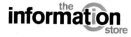

lowed a career in the Civil Service until, in 1991, she developed fibromyalgia, a chronic pain condition. Christine took up writing for therapeutic reasons and has, in the past few years, produced *Living with Fibromyalgia*, *The Fibromyalgia Healing Diet*, *The Chronic Fatigue Healing Diet*, *Coping with Polycystic Ovary Syndrome*, *Coping with Gout*, *How to Beat Pain* and *Coping with Eating Disorders and Body Image* (all published by Sheldon Press). She also writes for the Fibromyalgia Association UK and the related *FaMily* magazine. In recent years she has become interested in fiction writing, too.

Overcoming Common Problems Series

Selected titles
A full list of titles is available from Sheldon Press,
36 Causton Street, London SW1P 4ST, and on our website at
www.sheldonpress.co.uk

Assertiveness: Step by Step
Dr Windy Dryden and Daniel Constantinou

Breaking Free
Carolyn Ainscough and Kay Toon

Calm Down
Paul Hauck

Cataract: What You Need to Know
Mark Watts

Cider Vinegar
Margaret Hills

Comfort for Depression
Janet Horwood

Confidence Works
Gladeana McMahon

Coping Successfully with Pain
Neville Shone

Coping Successfully with Panic Attacks
Shirley Trickett

Coping Successfully with Period Problems
Mary-Claire Mason

Coping Successfully with Prostate Cancer
Dr Tom Smith

Coping Successfully with Ulcerative Colitis
Peter Cartwright

Coping Successfully with Your Hiatus Hernia
Dr Tom Smith

Coping Successfully with Your Irritable Bowel
Rosemary Nicol

Coping with Alopecia
Dr Nigel Hunt and Dr Sue McHale

Coping with Anxiety and Depression
Shirley Trickett

Coping with Blushing
Dr Robert Edelmann

Coping with Bowel Cancer
Dr Tom Smith

Coping with Brain Injury
Maggie Rich

Coping with Candida
Shirley Trickett

Coping with Chemotherapy
Dr Terry Priestman

Coping with Childhood Allergies
Jill Eckersley

Coping with Childhood Asthma
Jill Eckersley

Coping with Chronic Fatigue
Trudie Chalder

Coping with Coeliac Disease
Karen Brody

Coping with Cystitis
Caroline Clayton

Coping with Depression and Elation
Patrick McKeon

Coping with Down's Syndrome
Fiona Marshall

Coping with Dyspraxia
Jill Eckersley

Coping with Eating Disorders and Body Image
Christine Craggs-Hinton

Coping with Eczema
Dr Robert Youngson

Coping with Endometriosis
Jo Mears

Coping with Epilepsy
Fiona Marshall and
Dr Pamela Crawford

Coping with Fibroids
Mary-Claire Mason

Coping with Gout
Christine Craggs-Hinton

Coping with Heartburn and Reflux
Dr Tom Smith

Coping with Incontinence
Dr Joan Gomez

Coping with Long-Term Illness
Barbara Baker

Coping with Macular Degeneration
Dr Patricia Gilbert

Coping with the Menopause
Janet Horwood

Overcoming Common Problems Series

Overcoming Common Problems Series

Living with High Blood Pressure
Dr Tom Smith

Living with Hughes Syndrome
Triona Holden

Living with Loss and Grief
Julia Tugendhat

Living with Lupus
Philippa Pigache

Living with Nut Allergies
Karen Evennett

Living with Osteoarthritis
Dr Patricia Gilbert

Living with Osteoporosis
Dr Joan Gomez

Living with Rheumatoid Arthritis
Philippa Pigache

Living with Sjögren's Syndrome
Sue Dyson

Losing a Baby
Sarah Ewing

Losing a Child
Linda Hurcombe

Make Up or Break Up: Making the Most of Your Marriage
Mary Williams

Making Friends with Your Stepchildren
Rosemary Wells

Making Relationships Work
Alison Waines

Overcoming Anger
Dr Windy Dryden

Overcoming Anxiety
Dr Windy Dryden

Overcoming Back Pain
Dr Tom Smith

Overcoming Depression
Dr Windy Dryden and Sarah Opie

Overcoming Impotence
Mary Williams

Overcoming Jealousy
Dr Windy Dryden

Overcoming Loneliness and Making Friends
Márianna Csóti

Overcoming Procrastination
Dr Windy Dryden

Overcoming Shame
Dr Windy Dryden

Rheumatoid Arthritis
Mary-Claire Mason and Dr Elaine Smith

Shift Your Thinking, Change Your Life
Mo Shapiro

Stress at Work
Mary Hartley

Ten Steps to Positive Living
Dr Windy Dryden

The Assertiveness Handbook
Mary Hartley

The Candida Diet Book
Karen Brody

The Chronic Fatigue Healing Diet
Christine Craggs-Hinton

The Fibromyalgia Healing Diet
Christine Craggs-Hinton

The Irritable Bowel Diet Book
Rosemary Nicol

The PMS Diet Book
Karen Evennett

The Self-Esteem Journal
Alison Waines

The Traveller's Good Health Guide
Ted Lankester

Think Your Way to Happiness
Dr Windy Dryden and Jack Gordon

Treating Arthritis – The Drug-Free Way
Margaret Hills

Treating Arthritis – More Ways to a Drug-Free Life
Margaret Hills

Treating Arthritis Diet Book
Margaret Hills

Treating Arthritis Exercise Book
Margaret Hills and Janet Horwood

Understanding Obsessions and Compulsions
Dr Frank Tallis

When Someone You Love Has Depression
Barbara Baker

Your Man's Health
Fiona Marshall

Overcoming Common Problems

Living with Multiple Sclerosis

Christine Craggs-Hinton

sheldon **PRESS**

First published in Great Britain in 2006

Sheldon Press
36 Causton Street
London SW1P 4ST

The author and publisher have made every effort to ensure
that the external website and email addresses included in this book are
correct and up to date at the time of going to press. The author
and publisher are not responsible for the content, quality or
continuing accessibility of the sites.

British Library Cataloguing-in-Publication Data

A catalogue record for this book is available from the British Library

ISBN-13: 978–0–85969–982–2
ISBN-10: 0–85969–982–X

1 3 5 7 9 10 8 6 4 2

Typeset by Deltatype Limited, Birkenhead, Merseyside
Printed in Great Britain by Ashford Colour Press

I would like to dedicate this book to all the men and women who cope with MS every day. May you find the strength to accept the presence of MS in your life and to get pleasure from as many things as possible.

Contents

Acknowledgements

I would like to thank the following women – all of whom have MS – for helping me understand the condition and for allowing me to ask the most intimate of questions. I was struck by the spirit and determination shared by all three. They have learned, for the most part, to do whatever it takes to get the most out of life. I found their positive attitudes truly inspirational.

Sarah Elizabeth (Beth) Shea – Thanks to the wonders of email, Beth, a cousin who lives in Nova Scotia, gladly answered my numerous questions. It was she who gave me my first real insight into life with MS and the fortitude shown by many sufferers. Her own strength of character shone as clear as day across the miles.

Doreen Berrie-Barker – Despite numerous other problems in her life, and being in the clutches of a relapse when I spoke to her, Doreen was only too willing to help me to understand how she is affected by MS. I have found her spirit and courage remarkable and know that one day very soon her dream will come true.

Marysia Hibbert – Marysia is another lovely lady with a heart big enough for her to look outwards more than in. She was only too keen to answer my questions, and to give me a snapshot of her life with MS. If a positive attitude alone could bring you all you wished for, Marysia would have it.

Introduction

No one would deny that living with MS is a challenge. It's the challenge of a lifetime – not only for the person concerned, but also for family and friends. Indeed, in the early days, family and friends undergo similar emotions to those experienced by the person concerned, including anger, frustration, resentment and fear. Fortunately, at some point, most people with MS realize that their life is not over – not by any means. They recognize that they can continue to function, albeit with help on occasion; they can still get pleasure out of life, be of use to others, and make others happy. The trick is to be open to doing the things that make you feel good about yourself, whether that means new hobbies and interests, new skills, or even changing your career.

You may think that it is necessary to succeed in a venture of some kind to feel really good about yourself, but that's just not true. Positive feelings can come from something as simple as paying more attention to your loved ones, giving some of your time to good causes and so on. The positive feelings produced are then likely to be further enhanced by the very nature of MS, for it is a disease capable of throwing up a multitude of problems, different in every person. As a result of having little choice but to cope with these problems, you are likely to become a calmer, more rational person who refuses to let the little things get you down. So, MS is not a sentence to a life of misery and despair. Of course, it is hardly a good thing – not in a million years, and there is more depression related to MS than in the general population. However, people with MS tend to develop a strength of character missing in a lot of other people. And most learn to get a great deal from their lives.

Getting back to depression, it is only natural to feel miserable when hit with a relapse, but most people feel brighter once the relapse is behind them. When left with a new, permanent symptom, most learn gradually to integrate it into their unique personality. And then, once again, they lift up their heads and get on with their lives.

Reading this book should help you to move forward. It contains matter-of-fact information about MS – and knowledge takes away a lot of the fear. It also outlines the theories on the causes of MS; gives details about possible symptoms; and offers information on drug therapy, diet, occupational therapy, pregnancy and complementary therapies.

Get reading, find out the best and the worst of the situation, tell yourself it is OK to feel afraid, frustrated and angry at times, then get on with making the most of your future.

1

Multiple sclerosis – an overview

You are probably only too aware that multiple sclerosis (MS) can lead to severe debility, with people ending up in wheelchairs, and a multitude of disabling symptoms. What you may not realize, though, is that the disease progression is slow in most people. In fact, three-quarters of those with MS don't ever need to use a wheelchair, and those who do often find that it gives them greater freedom to get on with their lives.

As yet, the cause of MS has not been pinpointed, and we know it cannot be prevented or cured. However, a great deal of progress is being made in identifying the triggering mechanisms. As a result of recent research, we now have a variety of strategies that can greatly enhance the quality of life of people who have MS. These include the following:

- Drugs that can modify the course of the condition.
- Drugs that can reduce the length and severity of relapses.
- Strategies to help the person to manage their symptoms.
- Strategies to improve safety.
- Strategies to help the person get the most out of life.

So what exactly is MS?

MS was first described in Holland by a fourteenth-century doctor. It is an unpredictable inflammatory disease that primarily afflicts young adults. Its severity can range from mild to completely devastating, although only a few end up so disabled that they are unable to function. As the individual expression of the disease is as unique as our fingerprints, no two people with MS experience the same symptoms. The course of the disease can vary in the following ways:

- Timing – that is, the speed at which the disease progresses.
- Location – that is, the areas of the body attacked by MS.
- Severity – that is, the intensity of symptoms.

It is believed that MS can only arise in a person with a genetically damaged immune system. Such an immune system is unable to distinguish between proteins that originate from the body's own myelin – the substance that protects nerve cells – and proteins from invading viruses. As a result, it mistakenly produces antibodies that attack and destroy myelin. The body is thus allergic to itself, a condition referred to as 'autoimmunity'. Indeed, MS is considered an autoimmune disease, as you may already know.

Neurological involvement

In MS, the nerves of the central nervous system (CNS) – that is, the brain and spinal cord – slowly degenerate, so it is also a neurological disorder. The condition is characterized by the presence of multiple patches of abnormally hardened connective tissue called lesions or sclerosis – hence the term 'multiple sclerosis' – that are scattered irregularly throughout the central nervous system, but that exist mainly in the optic nerve, brainstem, spinal cord, white matter and cerebellum (the part of the brain at the back of the skull that co-ordinates and regulates muscular activity). We have all heard about the 'grey matter' of the brain – well, *white* matter regions are responsible for communication between the areas of grey matter and the rest of the body. Both types of brain matter are made up of nerve cells and both types can develop lesions.

When lesions begin to form, nerve impulses are transmitted inefficiently. The unfortunate result is gradual cognitive or muscular impairment.

A catch-all term

The name 'multiple sclerosis' has evolved as a catch-all term for chronic demyelination – degeneration of myelin – when the exact cause cannot be isolated.

Chronic demyelination can also be caused by a particular bacterial infection, but because the cause is known, the condition is given its own name – Lyme Disease – rather than being lumped in with MS. Chronic demyelination can also occur in a rare condition called chronic rubella encephalitis, but because we know the process is triggered by the measles vaccination, again the disease has a separate name.

The symptoms of MS

When we take a shower, operate a computer keyboard, or even scratch our heads, hundreds or thousands of central nervous system nerves are communicating effectively with hundreds or thousands of nerves in the peripheral nervous system (PNS) – which operates outside the brain and spinal cord. We depend on full and smooth functioning of both the central nervous system and peripheral nervous system for every movement we make, simple or complex. But when the immune system creates damage (lesions) within the central nervous system, as in MS, problems can run through the whole system.

The early symptoms of MS are likely to include numbness, pins and needles, involuntary eye movements, blurred or double vision, red–green colour distortion, tremor of the limbs, and bladder control problems. Subsequent symptoms can include more prominent motor problems such as muscle weakness in the limbs, unsteady gait, poor co-ordination, dizziness, fatigue, depression, short-term memory problems, difficulty concentrating, spasticity – excessive muscle contraction and an increased resistance to being stretched – muscle spasms, cramps, pain, partial or complete paralysis, tremors, hearing loss, blindness in one eye, incontinence, constipation, slurred speech, male impotence, problems in swallowing and an inability to control breathing. The latter two symptoms are rare.

The disease is largely marked by periods of progression, remission and relapse:

- Progression refers to the gradual advancement of the disease as it moves (usually very slowly) from one stage to another.
- Remission is the period during which symptoms are reduced, and often greatly eased. It can be short-lived, or persist for many years.
- A relapse is a period of exacerbated symptoms. Such symptoms can persist for between 24 hours and four weeks. It is also common to experience a temporary deterioration as a result of the onset of flu, a bladder infection and so on, but these things don't necessarily mean a relapse is under way. Factors known to

precipitate a relapse include emotional stress and psychological trauma, including shock, grief, anger, suppressed anger, rejection, humiliation, disappointment in love or career, and so on. Physical trauma can also bring on a relapse.

Progression, remission and relapse are discussed in more detail later on.

What causes MS?

Until the cause of MS is known, finding a cure is not possible. This is made more difficult because there appears to be a whole host of factors that can trigger the disease. The main trigger is believed to be dietary in nature (see Chapter 7). Other possible triggers include viruses and bacteria, vaccinations, trauma, stress, heavy metals and the inhalation of toxic chemicals (see Chapter 8). However, research indicates that MS can only be triggered in a person who carries the MS gene and therefore has a genetically damaged immune system. An estimated 5 per cent of northern Europeans carry the gene, but many of these people go through their lives disease-free.

Scientists have now established much of what happens within a susceptible body when a trigger has occurred. Primarily, the immune system mounts an attack on the body's own tissues, sending a far greater number of immune cells than normal into the central nervous system – the presence of large numbers of immune cells is called inflammation. The immune cells work very quickly to damage and destroy the myelin sheaths that protect the nerves.

Myelin degeneration

Brain matter (the central nervous system) is packed with nerve cells, each one of which is protected by a fatty white insulating substance called myelin. Myelin is essential as it improves the conduction of electrical impulses that travel along the nerves, and prevents electrical signals from leaking out. Myelin is also important for maintaining the health of the nerves. Because of its colour, myelin is often referred to as the 'white matter' of the brain and spinal cord. In MS, inflammation causes the myelin to break down and eventually be absorbed by the body – a process called 'demyelination'.

When nerves are stripped of their myelin protective coating, they fail to function efficiently, causing a wide range of symptoms. In time, as the disease progresses, the nerves themselves can become damaged. Symptoms depend on the site of the lesions within the central nervous system. Study of MRI scans has shown that the vast majority of lesions do not produce symptoms (Poser, 1986). This would appear to be due to other parts of the central nervous system taking over the functions previously carried out by the damaged nerves.

Researchers have also found evidence that the body attempts to correct myelin loss. For example, an increase in the density of the sodium channels, which carry electric charges, has been seen, and this enables the nerve cells to continue to communicate. The nerves also retain some capacity to restore their myelin protection. Such corrective processes are believed to be responsible for the remissions experienced by most MS patients. Sadly, though, the disease process nearly always outpaces these corrective actions, given time.

Inflammation

It is only when patches of inflammation – large numbers of immune cells – arise in the central nervous system that myelin can be attacked and broken down. The inflammation appears to occur as a result of irregularities in the immune system, which is the body's highly organized defender. If triggered into action by an aggressor such as a virus, the immune system mounts a defensive action that identifies and attacks the invader and then withdraws.

In MS, researchers believe that a virus or abnormal gene causes either myelin or the immune system to be faulty, as a result of which the immune system perceives myelin as an invader and attacks it. As stated, myelin is capable of repair, but often not all of it regenerates and some nerves are stripped bare of their protection. Scarring occurs at the site, and waste material is deposited into the scars. This is the process by which lesions or plaques are formed.

'T'-cell' activation – the autoimmune response

In MS, the autoimmune response is set into action when the immune system's major cells – called 'T-cells' – detect a foreign substance such as a virus, bacteria or other unidentified agent. Antibodies to

5

T-cells can always be found in MS, which means the T-cells are permanently on guard in readiness to command a battle. As soon as the T-cells detect what they interpret as a foreign substance, they give a command to the immune system, which prepares its antibodies for a fight.

In some people with MS, structures that mimic a component of myelin enter the circulatory system where they are quickly detected by the T-cells. These cells give commands to the immune system, and because it cannot differentiate between the foreign structures and the components of true myelin, the immune system begins to mistakenly attack its own cells.

The Epstein-Barr virus, herpes simplex, human papilloma virus, some flu viruses and a bacterial peptide called pseudomonas aeruginosa have a structural similarity to a component of myelin. They therefore also have the ability to activate T-cells.

The blood-brain barrier

Activated T-cells must enter the central nervous system before being able to command an attack. The central nervous system is the most important control unit in the body and is protected by a careful filtering mechanism – the 'blood–brain barrier' that employs the immune system when it detects a virus, bacteria or other foreign body entering the central nervous system. In MS, there are two different processes whereby the blood-brain barrier is breached and the immune system is confused into attacking healthy self-tissue (Herndon *et al.*, 1985). They are as follows:

- When the proteins in certain foods are very similar to proteins that occur naturally in the body, the immune system is unable to tell them apart and ends up attacking the body's own myelin, as well as the food proteins.
- When a process known as 'leaky gut syndrome' allows undigested food to enter the circulation, the immune system responds by attacking the invaders.

Can MS be inherited?

Researchers are coming to the conclusion that all autoimmune diseases are basically the result of the same genetic error. A 2001 study found, for example, that the T-cell antibodies in Type 1 diabetes are also confused by food proteins. Both diseases have been associated with cows' milk protein, but it is not known why the diseases develop in different locations and cause separate disorders.

Eskimos (Inuit), European gypsies and African Bantu – people who largely live in isolation – essentially do not develop MS, while native Indians of North and South America, Japanese and other Asian groups have a low incidence of the disease. The population of north-east Scotland has been seen, in one study, to have one of the highest incidence rates of MS in the world. Interestingly, 80 per cent of MS patients here share the same genetic marker (Francis *et al.*, 1987). More population studies are currently under way.

Within the general population, a person has less than a 1 per cent chance of contracting MS. However, the likelihood increases when a first-degree relative has the disease. A sibling, parent or child of a person with MS stands a 1–3 per cent chance of developing the disease; the identical twin of a person with MS stands a 30 per cent chance, but there is only a 4 per cent chance of a non-identical twin developing the disease if the other twin has it. First-degree relatives of MS patients are at a risk that is 20 to 50 times higher than that of the general population, but that is still only an overall risk of less than 5 per cent (Larner *et al.*, 1986). One study found a significant association between siblings with MS and a specific form of the disease, either relapsing-remitting or chronic progressive, but no association with the age of onset or severity of initial symptoms.

It is interesting that people who have lived the first 15 years of their lives between the fortieth and fiftieth degree of latitude in either hemisphere have been seen to be at greater risk of developing MS, and the risk remains permanent, regardless of whether they move to sunnier climes after the age of 15.

What course does MS generally take?

MS can progress in a variety of ways, and each course has relapses (also referred to as exacerbations, flare-ups or attacks) in common. The disease generally begins with a flare-up of acute or sub-acute neurological abnormalities such as numbness, tingling, double vision, bladder control problems, muscle weakness and so on. The relapse may be brief, or it may last a few months or even years.

Experts say that your general condition 15 years after the onset of MS gives a rough guide to your future condition.

Most people with MS – about 85 per cent – begin with the relapsing-remitting pattern of MS (see below).

Relapsing-remitting MS

Relapsing-remitting MS (RR-MS) usually occurs in younger people and is the most common form of the disease. People experience episodes of sudden deterioration during which new symptoms can appear and old ones resurface or worsen, followed by complete, or almost complete, alleviation of symptoms:

- Symptoms generally flare up for several days. They are fairly mild in 50 per cent of cases.
- The disease then goes into remission, during which time the symptoms either improve or disappear. Remissions may be spontaneous, or induced by immunosuppressive drugs.
- Someone who thinks she is in remission can have subtle attacks and not realize it. For example, her gait may be a little awkward or her hands a little numb for a few days.
- Remissions are almost always followed by relapses or periods of deteriorating ability.

Studies suggest that twice as many women as men have the RR variant of MS. A person will typically develop this form of MS in their twenties or thirties, although much later onset is known.

Benign MS

Benign MS is a term used to describe the disease in people with a diagnosis of RR-MS, but who experience it in a mild form, with negligible neurological symptoms and no serious or continuing disability. The disease may be simply an inconvenience at times, causing very little disturbance to the individual's life. Some people fail to suspect anything wrong throughout their lifetime, yet a post-mortem examination can reveal many central nervous system lesions.

Doctors believe that use of the term 'benign MS' should be discouraged as less than 5 per cent of the MS population suffer from this variant.

Progressive MS

Up to 70 per cent of RR-MS people eventually move into the progressive stage of the disease (Sibley, 1985), remissions gradually becoming fewer with less and less improvement. This is called secondary progressive MS (SP-MS). Once in this form, the disease generally takes a downhill course, but its severity varies widely. In some cases, the decline in physical abilities frequently seems to stop and minor relief is experienced. In other cases, people fail to experience any lessening of symptoms at all.

Because lesions now appear in the spinal cord rather than the brain, this phase of the disease causes abnormal bladder and bowel problems, and sexual dysfunction. Walking and balance problems are likely to arise too, and the person may eventually be confined to a wheelchair, and possibly at a much later stage to bed.

A small number of people are thrown straight into progressive MS without RR-MS arising first – this is called primary progressive MS (PP-MS). Men are as likely to develop this variant as women and the average age of onset is the late thirties and early forties.

Progressive-relapsing MS

This variant is characterized by a disease pattern that steadily worsens from the start. People with progressive-relapsing MS (PR-MS) face acute relapses, often with significant rallying, but sometimes with little recovery at all. Progressive-relapsing MS is relatively rare, with a frequency of only 5 per cent.

Malignant MS

Malignant MS is also known as Acute Multiple Sclerosis or Marburg's Variant. It describes a pattern whereby the disease moves forward rapidly, causing severe disability within a relatively short period of time. Fortunately, malignant MS is extremely rare.

Who gets MS?

MS is a leading cause of disability, with 1.1 million people worldwide having the disease. Most people experience their first symptoms between the ages of 20 and 40, with a peak incidence at between 20 and 30 years old. However, the disease has been diagnosed as early as the age of 15 and as late as 60. MS is twice as likely to occur in Caucasians (white race people) than in any other group. Indeed, populations of northern European ancestry are most likely to develop it, especially those of Scottish descent. MS is extremely rare among people with Asian, African and Hispanic backgrounds, but they are not immune.

The disease affects two to three times more females than males, and women are twice as likely as men to develop MS earlier in life. Later in life, the occurrence of the disease in men and women is almost equal. This would suggest a hormonal component to the disease process, women being more susceptible during their menstrual years. Males are more likely than women to develop primary progressive MS, while females tend to experience more relapses.

MS is more prevalent in the more temperate regions of the world, more so than in the tropics. The highest incidence is in northern Europe, southern Australia and the middle regions of North America. The number of cases is rising in southern Europe, however, but it is not known whether this is due to environmental factors or genetics.

A family history of MS puts a person at a small risk of 2–4 per cent.

What is the long-term outlook for someone with MS?

Although MS is not a fatal disease, it can present life-threatening risks in severe cases. Furthermore, for the majority of people with MS, the emotional impact of the disease is substantial. Studies indicate that women stay more positive than men, and that men are more likely to develop depressive illness. The severity of the disease varies considerably from person to person, and the course is unpredictable.

Between 10 and 30 per cent of people with MS have a very mild form of it. They may have little or no disability, and a normal life expectancy. People who suffer only from optic neuritis (see Chapter 2) and symptoms that affect the senses have a better prognosis than do people with more widespread symptoms.

An important 2000 study used a scale called the Kurtzke Disability Status Scale to predict disability in MS (see the table opposite).

The Kurtzke Disability Status Scale for MS

1 No disability and minimal neurological problems.

2 Minimal disability. There is likely to be either slight weakness and fatigue, stiffness, mild disturbance of gait or mild visual disturbance.

3 Moderate disability. This person has monoparesis (partial or incomplete paralysis affecting one or part of one extremity) or mild hemiparesis (slight paralysis affecting one side of the body). Symptoms also include moderate ataxia (the loss of full control of bodily movements), disturbing sensory loss (such as poor memory, poor concentration, mood swings and so on), or prominent bladder or eye symptoms. There may be a combination of several of these symptoms, to a less serious degree.

4 Relatively severe disability. Despite considerable problems, this person is self-sufficient, able to walk unaided, able to be up and about for 12 hours a day, able to go to work and to carry on normal living activities, with the exception of maintaining a healthy sex life.

5 Disability severe enough to preclude working. However, this person can walk unaided for up to 500 metres.

6 Needs assistance walking, for example a cane, crutches, or braces.

7 Essentially restricted to a wheelchair, but able to wheel oneself and enter and leave the chair without assistance.

8 Essentially restricted to bed or a chair. However, this person retains many self-care functions and has effective use of his or her arms.

9 Helpless and bedridden.

10 Death due to MS, resulting from respiratory paralysis, coma of uncertain origin, or following repeated or prolonged epileptic seizures.

The study indicated that in people with relapsing-remitting MS, progression to moderate disability is often very slow, compared with patients with other forms of the disease. Once a person reaches a score of 4 on the scale, the disease worsens at the same rate in people with all forms of the disease.

Please remember that the vast majority of people remain able to function, albeit with assistance in some cases. Only a small percentage of sufferers develop such severe disability that they fall into categories 5 to 10, as outlined in the table on page 11.

Infections

There is evidence that central nervous system inflammation in MS can be caused by an upper respiratory tract infection, such as a cold or flu, and also from gastroenteritis. The inflammation has the effect of triggering a relapse, with the appearance of new neurological symptoms or the significant worsening of existing neurological symptoms.

Due to increased immune system activity, MS symptoms almost certainly worsen when a person has a cold or flu. Indeed, a viral infection is the most frequent event to precede a relapse. In one study, 8 per cent of all relapses were related to a viral infection. Whether the flu jab is safe in MS is still a matter for debate. Until better advice comes along, it is recommended that you have it only if it is deemed absolutely necessary.

2

Possible symptoms of MS

With MS there is no way of knowing what long-term problems will arise, if any. Each case of MS is very different, and what affects one person will not necessarily affect another. It all depends on the areas in the central nervous system in which lesions develop.

Visual problems

Visual symptoms are fairly common in MS, but seldom result in blindness. When the nerves that control an eye are affected, a variety of eye disorders can arise. These include optic neuritis, double vision and uncontrollable eye movements.

Optic neuritis

Eye pain – optic neuritis – is caused by inflammation of the optic nerve or the presence of lesions along the pathways that control eye movements and visual co-ordination. When inflammation is the cause, the problem is usually temporary, arising most frequently during a relapse. However, lesions can mean permanent damage, and therefore permanent symptoms.

Optic neuritis is characterized by a sharp pain when moving one eye – it is rare that both eyes are affected at the same time. The eyeballs may feel sensitive and there is usually an accompanying headache, with resulting blurred or greying of the vision, or even blindness in one eye. In some cases, a scotoma or dark spot is present in the middle of the visual field. Any loss of vision rarely lasts for more than a few days. If blindness persists, you may be offered treatment with intravenous steroids such as methylpredniso-lone, followed by a short course of oral steroids. The outcome has been shown in studies to be more encouraging with steroid treatment than with no treatment at all. The problems generally resolve within four to twelve weeks.

It is estimated that 55 per cent of people with MS experience at least one episode of optic neuritis – often the first symptom of MS, it can exist just as pain rather than a combination of pain and visual problems. Note that not everyone who experiences optic neuritis is developing MS.

Double vision

Also called diplopia, double vision arises when the muscles controlling the movements of each eye are not exactly co-ordinated, normally due to weakness.

If the problem fails to resolve itself – it normally does – a short course of corticosteroids may be needed. In severe cases, it may be helpful to wear a patch over one eye for driving, reading and so on. However, patching is not recommended for long periods as it slows the brain's ability to interpret double vision.

Numbness

Numbness in the face and body or arms and legs is one of the most common MS symptoms. It can feel slightly uncomfortable, or so severe that it reduces your ability to use the affected area. For example, very numb fingers can make it impossible to get dressed, washed, write or use a keyboard, and very numb feet can make it impossible to walk or drive a car.

Numbness often occurs in the build-up to a relapse, and it is likely to be one of the main problems when the relapse is under way.

Keeping safe

When you have severe numbness in your face, eating can be difficult. There's a risk of biting your tongue or the inside of your mouth. You should, therefore, try to eat as slowly and carefully as possible. Numbness in other parts of your body signals the need for you to be careful near fires, hot water and other sources of heat – you could burn without realizing it.

There are no medications to treat numbness, but it is generally not disabling and should resolve when the relapse ends.

Fatigue

This symptom is believed to be the most common MS problem, affecting 80 per cent of people with MS at some stage. Fatigue can either be mild, or so severe that it is difficult to function. It can be

14

the most prominent symptom in some people – often those with minimal disability – and can either be physical or mental, or both. Fatigue can be divided into:

- Physical fatigue – feelings of weariness, lassitude and lack of energy. It may be accompanied by nausea.
- Mental fatigue – poor concentration, difficulty in making decisions, feeling tired all the time, the feeling that your thought processes are churning through treacle. The mental fatigue of MS is not connected with depression, even though the two may coexist. However, your family, friends and work colleagues may interpret it as depression, or even as lack of effort.

The fatigue of MS is different in several ways from that experienced by a healthy person:

- It is generally more severe than normal fatigue.
- It is usually present on a daily basis.
- It arises far more easily.
- It can appear after a normal activity, like going to the shop or doing the ironing.
- It is just as likely to occur after a good night's sleep.
- It tends to be heightened as the day advances.
- It is often worsened by heat and humidity.
- It is more likely than normal fatigue to handicap daily functioning.

In MS, fatigue can be caused by inactivity – when the muscles are out of condition, or it can be a side-effect of another medical condition, such as anaemia or thyroid disorder, both of which are treatable. If your fatigue is deemed to not be a result of a coexisting condition, your doctor may refer you for one or more of the following:

- Occupational therapy, so you are more easily able to perform tasks at home and at work.
- Physical therapy, to find more energy-efficient ways of walking and carrying out other activities.
- Psychological help, such as learning stress-management techniques and how to pace yourself effectively. You will be shown how to relax, and possibly offered psychotherapy.

- To get you over a particularly bad patch, you may also be prescribed short-term medications to help you to sleep.

Unfortunately, few studies have been conducted to determine the best treatments for the fatigue associated with MS. Modafinil (Provigil and Alertec) is a new drug that promotes long-lasting wakefulness. It is taken in the morning and doesn't seem to disturb normal night-time sleep. Studies suggest that amantadine (Symmetrel) may also be helpful. Pemoline (Cylert) is a common treatment for fatigue, but evidence suggests it is no better than a placebo and has considerable side-effects.

Bladder problems

According to studies, between 80 and 90 per cent of people with MS experience bladder problems, because MS lesions block or delay the transmission of nerve signals in areas of the central nervous system that control the bladder and urinary sphincter. The sphincter is the muscle surrounding the opening of the bladder. It controls the storage and flow of urine and opens to let urine out. Voluntary control over urination comes via this muscle.

Bladder dysfunction can be signalled by the following:

- The need to urinate frequently, usually with urgency.
- Hesitancy in starting the flow of urine.
- Frequently getting up in the night to urinate.
- The inability to hold urine in the bladder.
- Failure of the bladder to empty properly.

The above symptoms may be the result of a 'spastic' bladder – one that is unable to hold the normal amount of urine, or is unable to empty properly or always retains some urine in it. The latter can lead to urinary tract infections.

Of course, having an untreated bladder problem cannot only cause personal hygiene concerns; it can also interfere with normal living and socializing. There are also emotional implications, for it feels neither feminine/masculine nor sexy to be dashing to the loo every few minutes. For those who resort to wearing incontinence pads, it is common to feel worthless and ashamed.

Treatment

The aim of medication is to improve quality of life, reduce the likelihood of urinary tract infections – these can exacerbate other MS symptoms – and encourage bladder control. The problem can often be managed by medication. However, in severe cases, when it is impossible to empty the bladder, occasional self-catheterization may be required. In such instances, a small tube is inserted into the bladder to release the urine, and can be done whenever convenient throughout the day. With training and the support of a health care professional, most people can master the technique.

In cases where self-catheterization is not possible, a long-term indwelling catheter may be the best option.

Treating urge incontinence

Urge incontinence (the need to urinate frequently) is common in MS. To minimize social difficulties, it is recommended that you don't drink fluids before going to places where toilets are not easily available. When possible, you should urinate every three to four hours. A number of medications are available for the treatment of urge incontinence, including anticholinergic drugs such as propantheline bromine (Pro-Banthine), tolterodine (Detrol), or oxybutynin (Ditropan). The use of Botulinum toxin – a purified substance derived from bacteria, used to block the nerve signal from the nerve to the muscle – injected into the urinary tract muscles is also being investigated.

Stimulation of the sacral nerve – InterStim – is also proving beneficial. The electrical pulses help to retrain nerves in the pelvic area.

Treating urinary retention

Urinary retention, where some urine is held back in the bladder, occurs in some people with MS, as stated. However, it is possible for urination to be stimulated by applying gentle but firm pressure to the bladder area with the fist or hand, by tapping against it, or by straining. The drugs being tried with some success for this problem are desmopressin (DDAVP) – ordinarily used for bed-wetting in children – and maprotiline (Ludiomil), an antidepressant. If neither pressure, tapping, straining nor medication do the trick, self-catheterization may be needed intermittently. When it is impossible to self-catheterize, an indwelling catheter may need to be placed in the urinary tract.

New surgical procedures that either reconstruct the bladder or divert the flow of urine may be the best option in severe cases of bladder dysfunction. Note, though, that urinary symptoms remain intermittent for years in the majority of cases; therefore, for as long as possible, treatment approaches should be limited to medications and other reversible therapies.

Treating urinary tract infections

Urinary tract infection (UTI) is common in MS and includes pain on urination, increased urgency to urinate, and a rise in the number of times you need to dash to the loo. When you experience any MS symptom flare-ups or a change in bladder symptoms, your urine should be analysed in a laboratory. Treatment of urinary tract infection is based on antibiotic regimes. You can help yourself, however, by drinking plenty of cranberry juice. Many women have known for a long time that cranberry juice is good for treating urinary tract problems. A recent study confirmed this, with the women in the study drinking 50 ml (about 2 oz) of cranberry juice daily.

Bowel problems

A number of bowel problems can be experienced by people with MS. The most common is constipation, characterized by the production of hard, pellet-like stools and difficulty with complete emptying of the bowel. With constipation, bowel incontinence can sometimes occur, usually after a few days without a bowel movement. In this instance, the colon or rectum becomes irritated and a runny stool leaks around the blockage.

Constipation or incontinence can be a result of the following:

- The 'gastro-colic reflex' – the normal urge to empty your bowels – can become weakened.
- The movement of food through the digestive tract can become mal-coordinated or slowed.
- There may be loss of sensation in the anorectal area, decreasing the normal urge to empty your bowels.

- The rectum can be spastic and therefore not able to open properly to allow the stool to pass.
- A lack of mobility in the person, perhaps if they sit down all day, can cause bowel dysfunction.
- A loss of muscle tone in the abdominal wall can allow the colon to become larger, and so decrease transit time of food through the digestive tract.
- Many of the medications used to treat spasticity, bladder spasms and other MS symptoms can cause constipation as a side-effect.

Bowel problems cause not only discomfort, but also feelings of shame, humiliation and worthlessness. The best treatments are things you can do for yourself, like the following:

- Drink plenty of water – at least 6–8 glasses a day.
- Ensure there is lots of fibre in your diet. As well as helping to keep you regular, a high-fibre diet lowers cholesterol and decreases the risk of bowel or colon cancer. For breakfast, eat bran flakes, Raisin Bran or All-Bran. During the rest of the day, eat plenty of fruit and vegetables. Your bread, cereal and pasta foods should be wholegrain. If you are unable to eat whole grains as well as fruit and vegetables, ask your doctor or chemist about the possibility of your taking a fibre supplement.
- Try to get into the habit of going to the toilet at a regular time every day. After breakfast or your mid-morning cup of tea or coffee are the best times of all. Often sitting there reading a book, perhaps rubbing your stomach a little, will bring about the desired effect, even if the urge has eluded you. Sitting there for up to an hour every day can reduce the risk of your losing control later in the day.
- Take regular exercise, if possible. Regular exercise encourages the digestive system to operate more smoothly and can help to avoid the dependence on laxatives, enemas or colonic irrigation.

If your bowel problems persist, enemas and laxatives are still not your best option. They slow down the bowel and cause an imbalance in electrolytes, the substances that conduct electrical impulses from the nerves – the balance of electrolytes in our bodies is essential for the normal functioning of our cells and organs. Furthermore, the gut becomes used to enemas and laxatives and greater and greater doses are required to achieve the same effect. Laxatives can also cause painful stomach cramps. It is better to add a poorly absorbable sugar to the diet, such as lactulose (Chronulac), made up of glucose and fructose, or sorbitol, a low-calorie bulk sweetener. Both can react with other medications, so are available only on prescription. To get things going, however, you may need to use a fairly strong suppository such as bisacodyl (Correctol or Dulcolax) after breakfast. It is best to discuss treatment options with your doctor.

Spasticity

'Spasticity' is the name given to muscle stiffness and the spasms resulting from involuntary muscle contractions. The latter can manifest as sudden movements of the muscles, or as prolonged muscle contraction. One of the more common symptoms of MS, spasticity can range from an occasional feeling of tightening in the muscles to the experience of painful uncontrollable spasms of the limbs, usually the legs. As a result of the latter, the person can feel sapped and experience an increase in general fatigue. Tightness in and around the joints can also be a symptom of spasticity, and can create pain in the lower back.

There are two types of spasticity in MS, both more likely in the latter stages of the disease:

- Extensor spasms: when attempting to make a movement, the quadriceps (the muscles on the front of the thigh) can suddenly tighten and make the legs shoot out straight, locking very close together, often crossed over at the ankles. This looks and feels startling and usually happens at night, in bed. It is rarely painful, however. Tilting the head so the chin moves towards the chest generally breaks the spasm. Extensor spasms can arise in the arms as well.
- Flexor spasms: this type of spasticity is generally a later event, occurring in the chronic progressive phase of MS. The muscles involved are the hamstrings – the muscles on the back of the upper leg – that bend the leg at the knee and hip joints. Flexor spasms can occur when you are sitting, lying down or standing.

However, if you are standing, a flexor spasm will make you fall. The drug baclofen (Lioresal) works to blunt over-active reflexes and is usually helpful in treating this type of spasm.

Spasticity varies remarkably from person to person. The muscle tightening is likely to occur in the morning, after prolonged immobility, or in some cases even after sitting still for a minute or two. It is only on moving around, perhaps doing some stretching exercises, that you can slowly loosen up. When painful spasms occur on waking, getting out of bed can be very difficult. Some people hate going to bed at night because they have such problems in the morning.

Spasticity can be aggravated by heat, humidity and infections, and can be triggered by coughing, sneezing, hiccoughs or laughing. Tight clothing has even been known to be a trigger. Mild spasticity can actually help to improve muscle tone in the legs, which can be of great assistance when walking. However, this benefit can be lost when medications are taken. The best treatment for mild spasticity is regular exercise to improve strength and range of motion. This should take the form of daily stretching exercise, as well as mobility and strengthening exercise.

Your doctor or neurologist is likely to refer you for the relevant specialist treatment such as occupational therapy, physiotherapy, and pain rehabilitation. Nerve-end blocking or other surgical procedures may also be used, depending on the individual case.

There are a variety of drug therapies for treating spasticity. However, as some of them should not be used in pregnancy, you should tell your doctor if you are pregnant or planning to get pregnant. The drugs are as follows:

- Baclofen (Lioresal). This drug has long been the preferred treatment for moderate to severe spasticity. It can be taken orally or administered using an implanted pump; the latter method has shown great benefits. Possible side-effects include drowsiness, confusion and a rubbery sensation in the legs.
- Gabapentin (Neurontin). Developed to control seizures, this can be used in MS to reduce spasticity. Its other benefits include alleviating facial pain and improving vision. Possible side-effects include drowsiness, difficulty sleeping, changes in appetite, fluid retention and loss of co-ordination.

- Pregabalin (Lyrica). Another drug developed to reduce seizures, Lyrica is also used to treat spasticity, but at lower doses than gabapentin. Possible side-effects include blurred or double vision, cognitive problems (memory, concentration, etc.), tremor and vertigo.
- Diazepam (Valium). This can be used to treat both spasticity and anxiety, but, as time passes, it can take larger and larger dosages to achieve the same result. The possible side-effects include dizziness, drowsiness and confusion. People with severe clinical depression should not take diazepam.
- Botulinum toxin. Injections of botulinum toxin (Dysport) are being investigated as a treatment of spasticity in specific areas of the body. In a study carried out in the year 2000, the drug was reported to be beneficial in helping to ease hip spasticity in up to two-thirds of patients. It has no major side-effects.
- Dantrolene (Dantrium). This drug is often prescribed for MS patients who are unable to tolerate diazepam (Valium) or baclofen (Lioresal). However, because dantrolene causes muscle weakness, it is best suited for those who are wheelchair bound but still suffer from spasticity, or for those whose muscles are still strong. In each case, the drug-induced weakness shouldn't be unduly debilitating. The possible side-effects include nausea, vomiting and anorexia. Higher doses of this drug can lead to liver damage.
- Electrical stimulation applied directly to the spastic muscles is proving to be beneficial.

Surgery for spasticity

Surgery should be considered only in very severe cases, where medication and exercise are of no benefit at all. Surgery involves cutting the affected tendons, but won't completely eliminate spasticity in the affected area. However, it can result in the loss of some movement and sensation.

Stiffness

Stiffness in the joints is common in MS and can make walking very difficult, especially when combined with vertigo, fatigue, spasticity and/or mal-coordination. Affected fingers and hands are particularly hard to come to terms with. After all, our hands make thousands of small movements in a day, many of them necessary to our normal everyday functions and working lives.

When joint stiffness occurs, it is not worth forcing your body into action – indeed, the stiffness can worsen with movement. When the stiffness starts to ease, start to coax the affected area back into movement.

Gait

It's due to the nerves running the whole length of the spinal cord that our legs are able to move. In MS, lesions anywhere along the spinal cord can cause problems in the legs and so in walking. Regular exercise is beneficial for all gait problems, but your doctor should first be consulted. Your gait problems will then be evaluated by a medical professional, after which an appropriate therapy programme can be planned.

Challenges to walking and gait (the manner of walking) are as follows:

- Muscle weakness in one or both legs. This can cause problems such as toe drag and foot drop. However, a new electrical stimulator – called the Odstock Dropped Foot Stimulator – is showing promising results for correcting gait problems. It entails the use of a special kind of brace with a switch in the heel, worn by the person with MS. At intervals, the switch is turned on to help the toe pick up correctly – the impulses feel like pins and needles and are well tolerated by most people. This kind of stimulation is still experimental and not yet in general use.
- Balance and co-ordination problems. These cause a swaying or 'drunken' gait. When your gait is so unsteady you are in danger of falling or bumping into things, you would benefit greatly from the use of a stick, wheelchair or scooter.
- Numbness and tingling in the legs and feet. A person with numb feet, for example, will be unable to feel the floor or know where their feet are. They will therefore find it impossible to walk. When one foot is numb, walking may be possible with the help of a stick or crutches.

- Muscle tightness or spasticity (see the section above). Very tight muscles can greatly impede walking and stretching exercises may be prescribed.
- Fatigue. When fatigue is at its worst, a person with MS may not have sufficient strength for walking.

Many people believe that long-term walking problems arise in the progressive stages of MS. In truth, lesions can occur in any part of the central nervous system at any time. If you don't have progressive MS, any walking problems are likely to be temporary, and should be gone by the end of the relapse. Meanwhile, accept whatever assistance devices you need to get around more easily, and take advantage of a tailored programme to help improve your gait.

Vertigo and poor co-ordination

Dizziness and balance problems (known as vertigo) are common in MS. They cause some people to feel off-balance or lightheaded. Less often, there is the feeling that they or their surroundings are spinning, which can have a disastrous effect on their ability to walk and perform other activities. Like all MS symptoms, vertigo and poor co-ordination are a result of the development of lesions in the central nervous system – except in this instance the lesions are located in the myriad of pathways that synchronize the input required by the brain to create and maintain balance and stability.

The sensations of dizziness and mal-coordination can be short-lived, or persist for several weeks. People with MS describe it as a kind of dizziness that makes the ground seem to pitch and roll, as if they are sailing the high seas. Some people can feel very nauseous, and may even be sick; others are assailed by fatigue and weakness. When you are trying to walk with these problems, your legs can be poorly co-ordinated and the result is a clumsy, drunken gait. Using a stick can not only indicate to people that you are sober, it can also help you to walk better and give you the confidence to go out instead of staying indoors.

When vertigo becomes a problem or lasts a long time, you should see your doctor. Symptoms generally respond to anti-motion sickness drugs, anti-nausea treatment or skin patches that deliver scopolamine, a drug that depresses the central nervous system. In severe cases, a short course of corticosteroids may be prescribed.

Pain

Contrary to what was formerly believed, most people with MS suffer pain. Indeed, in one study, 55 per cent reported that they had experienced 'clinically significant pain' at some stage in their illness. In the same survey, 48 per cent were troubled by chronic pain. The pain spectrum seems to run from minor twinges and aches, which are common to most people, through to severe pain.

The 'primary' pain felt by people with MS is that which arises as a direct result of lesions that are present. It comes, therefore, from nerve sources and is termed 'neurogenic' or 'neuropathic'. It is primary pain that is discussed in this section.

Note that sudden-onset pain, or an intensifying of pain, does not indicate a worsening of MS.

Facial pain and symptoms related to spasm

Facial pain (usually trigeminal neuralgia) occurs in only 1–2 per cent of people with MS. When MS lesions cause the trigeminal nerve to be inflamed, the result is a cutting or burning pain on one side of the face, similar to toothache or earache. The pain can be constant or spasmodic, and is often triggered by eating or temperature extremes. It can be so intense it interferes with sleeping and eating.

If over-the-counter painkillers fail to alleviate facial pain, it can be treated effectively with anticonvulsive medications. Carbamazepine (Tegretol) is currently the drug of choice. (Carbamazepine is also of benefit in other types of MS pain and spasm-related symptoms, including itching and aching.) Another anti-seizure drug, gabapentin (Neurontin), however, may be particularly effective for MS. This drug also appears to improve the blurred vision associated with MS and may help spasticity in general. Other drugs used for this symptom include pregabalin (Lyrica), diazepam (Valium) and the antidepressant amitriptyline (Elavil). If these drugs fail to work, your doctor or neurologist may consider injecting alcohol into the nerve in order to numb it for a period.

If severe pain persists, some people elect to have a section of a nerve surgically blocked or removed. This relieves the pain, but causes a sensation of numbness. Before you commit to such a procedure, you should ask the doctor to temporarily block the nerve with an anaesthetic so you can experience the numbness before undergoing irreversible surgery.

Llermitte's paraesthesia

This is either a brief electric-shock type of pain or a sensation of tingling down the back and into the legs and arms. Because it is caused by bending your neck forward, the best treatment is to wear a soft surgical collar or simply to avoid bending your neck. Anticonvulsant medications are sometimes prescribed.

Pseudoradicular pain

Similar to sciatica, this is felt continuously in one leg, or in one part of the body or in an arm. It may either be experienced as icy coldness or burning heat. Unfortunately, the appropriate pain-relieving drugs have undesirable muscle weakness as a side-effect, making this condition difficult to treat.

Burning and aching around the body

Also neurological in origin, this 'girdling' type of pain varies in intensity and can be treated with the anticonvulsant gabapentin (Neurontin), or the newer pregabalin (Lyrica), which is effective at a lower dosage than gabapentin. Girdling pain can also be treated with antidepressants such as amitryptyline (Elavil) and imipramine (Tofranil) which modify the way that the central nervous system reacts to pain. Don't be worried about using anticonvulsants or antidepressants. Their anti-pain properties were discovered during their development, and now they are routinely prescribed for neuropathic pain.

Secondary pain

Secondary pain is so called because it arises from any stress and strain on the muscles, ligaments, joints and bones rather than directly from nerve sources. It is usually felt as aching in the hips, lower back, legs and arms. Being immobile for long periods before moving around can provoke the aching, as can poor sitting and walking postures.

Paracetamol or ibuprofen can normally control secondary pain. However, you may wish first to try using a warm compress on the affected area – a heated wheat bag feels good. For further advice on beating pain, see Chapter 4.

Depression

According to recent studies, clinical depression occurs more often in chronic disabling conditions than among the general population. A quarter of newly diagnosed people with MS suffer an episode of clinical depression as a reaction to the news, and depression continues to raise its ugly head as the disease progresses. It's important to note, however, that depression in no way suggests a weak character and should not be seen as something shameful that is best kept hidden. In recent years we have learned the following about depression:

- Sadness and low mood that comes and goes cannot be categorized as 'clinical depression' – the latter has continuous symptoms lasting two weeks or more, and is of a severity that disturbs daily living.
- It may be reactive – the result of stresses and difficult life situations. Any condition that brings feelings of frustration and irritation can provoke reactive depression. Reactive depression can also be clinical depression, given the above-mentioned severity.
- In MS, depression may also be caused by the disease process itself. If there is damage to myelin as well as the nerves that are involved with the emotions, a variety of behavioural changes may occur, and they include depression.
- The depression in MS may arise as a result of changes in the immune system and neuroendocrine systems – the systems in the body that fight invaders and control levels of chemicals. In MS, mood changes can be accompanied by changes in the immune system and altered chemical levels. Depression can be due to chemical imbalance alone.

- People who are severely disabled in MS don't necessarily suffer more from depression than those with milder symptoms.
- Studies have shown that people with MS are more prone to depression during a relapse.
- Drugs such as steroids can give rise to depression as a side-effect. Steroids are occasionally prescribed to treat a relapse.
- Sadly, the chances of experiencing suicidal feelings are greater in MS than in people who don't have the disease.

If you have MS, try to remember that depression is a worldwide problem, and that there are many diseases and disorders that increase the likelihood of depression arising other than MS. In the healthy population, depression is often caused by the stresses and strains of life, which can be substantial. Moreover, the general population is just as likely as the MS population to suffer depression as a result of a chemical imbalance.

Grieving

In the early days after MS is diagnosed, it is common not only for the person affected, but also for their partner, to be stricken with depression. The possibility of disability and loss of independence is difficult to adjust to, and a bout of depression is only to be expected, I'm afraid. It's the type of depression that comprises mainly grief, where future losses are mourned; for this reason, it is time-limited and usually resolves on its own. You should still find that you retain certain interests and enjoy some activities. However, when the depression is so intense that you are interested in nothing and feel unable to perform your usual activities, it has flipped over into 'clinical depression'.

Clinical depression

Clinical depression is characterized by major depressive episodes, and includes:

- Feelings of sadness.
- Being tearful, and crying for much of the time.
- Loss of energy.
- Lack of interest in things that were once pleasurable.
- Loss of appetite, or an increased appetite.
- Feeling agitated and irritated.

- Insomnia, or excessive sleeping.
- Fatigue and the slowing down of behaviour.
- Feelings of hopelessness or worthlessness.
- Decreased sex drive.
- Difficulty with thinking, concentration and making decisions.
- Unexplained aches and pains.
- Stomach ache and digestive problems.
- Thoughts of death or suicide, or planning your own death.

When people who are depressed withdraw from activities, their life becomes empty, creating a downward spiral. The situation is compounded by the fact that depression can cause relationship problems, work issues or family unrest. It is likely to need treatment from a medical professional for relationships to improve and for you to enjoy life again.

Getting help

The first step along the road to recovery from depression is to accept that you are depressed. The second step is to actively seek help. Taken together, these steps are often the most difficult part of the entire recovery process – but they are also the most important. When you go to your doctor, take a trusted friend or family member if that makes you feel more comfortable, and tell the doctor exactly how you have been feeling. There are numerous treatment options to help you get back on track. First of all, you are likely to be examined to ensure that your symptoms are not being caused by medications or another illness. You may then be prescribed a course of antidepressant drugs – there are several types available.

Tricyclic antidepressants may be of benefit to MS symptoms other than depression. Amitriptyline (Elavil), for example, can help to moderate the extreme mood swings that may occur in MS. These mood swings are sometimes referred to as 'emotional incontinence', meaning the person is unable to control his or her emotions. Mood swings can be more distressing than physical symptoms for some people. Other tricyclic antidepressants include desipramine (Norpramin, Pertofrane) and imipramine (Tofranil), which can also improve bladder symptoms in some people. Such drugs, however, are capable of producing severe side-effects. The newer drugs, known as SSRIs (serotonin-reuptake inhibitors), which include fluoxetine (Prozac), sertraline (Zoloft), and paroxetine (Seroxat or Paxil), may be better tolerated. Extreme side-effects, such as suicide and murderous thoughts, have been related to Prozac in a small number of people, but they are the exception rather than the rule. Prozac is the most widely used prescription antidepressant in the Western world and is of great benefit to many people. A study of sertraline (Zoloft) suggested that it may also moderate the immune system's inflammatory response. An antidepressant called Rolipram is also proving to have powerful anti-inflammatory effects. Studies on its benefits in MS are under way.

Antidepressants are most effective when used in conjunction with psychotherapy, which enlists the use of a variety of treatment techniques. During psychotherapy you speak with a licensed mental health care professional who helps you to identify and work through the factors that may be triggering the depression.

Warning signs of suicide

The following are the warning signs that may be given out by someone who is seriously contemplating suicide. If you recognize them in someone, contact a mental health professional immediately. If that's not possible, ring 999. Possible signs of impending suicide are:

- Talking about killing oneself.
- Always talking or thinking about death.
- Saying things like 'It would be better if I weren't here', and 'What point is there in going on?'
- Feeling hopeless and worthless.
- Depression that seems to be getting worse – that is, problems with sleeping and eating, and loss of interest in anything.
- Tempting fate by taking risks when driving and so on.
- Suddenly switching from being very sad to being unusually calm or appearing to be happy.
- Visiting or phoning people who are important to that person.
- Putting his or her affairs in order.

Tremors

Tremors, or uncontrollable shaking in various parts of the body, are fairly common in MS. They are caused by damage to the complex nerve pathways responsible for movement co-ordination.

There are several types of tremor, which include the following:

- Postural tremor, which occurs when you are sitting or standing, but not when you are lying down.
- Intention tremor. This is the most common type of tremor and can be the most disabling. Such tremors take place when you have been at rest, then you make a movement – reaching out, grasping, moving a hand or foot to a different position and so on.
- Nystagmus. This type of tremor comes in the form of jumpy eye movements.

Treatment of tremors

Tremors are notoriously difficult to treat, and drug therapy has been very disappointing. This includes anti-tuberculosis medications such as isoniazid (INH); the antihistamine hydroxyzine (Atarax and Vistaril); the beta-blocker propranolol (Inderal); the anticonvulsive primidone (Mysoline); a diuretic callec acetazolamide (Diamox); and anti-anxiety drugs such as buspirone (Buspar) and clonazepam (Klonopin).

Weight applied to the affected limb is beneficial in about 20 per cent of cases of postural and intention tremor.

The psychological impact of tremors

Tremor can have a very strong emotional impact on a person, and some affected people isolate themselves socially in order to avoid embarrassment. However, isolation often leads only to depression and further psychological problems. A psychologist or counsellor may be able to help you to be more comfortable in public. Talk to your doctor if you are finding it difficult to cope.

Cognitive dysfunction

Up to 65 per cent of people with MS develop some degree of cognitive impairment, even in the early stages of the disease when there is little or no physical disability – in fact, cognitive dysfunction can even be the first symptom. The word 'cognitive' refers to mental activities such as thinking, attention, remembering, information processing, learning and visuospatial awareness. However, studies have indicated that only 5–10 per cent of people with MS develop problems that are serious enough to interfere significantly with their daily activities. Language skills and intellectual ability are usually preserved.

Impairment of cognitive function can have a huge impact on the person's confidence and quality of life. Fatigue, depression, anxiety and stress can make cognitive problems appear worse, and so present a real challenge. The severity of cognitive dysfunction varies widely among people with MS. For example, in studies of memory, 40 per cent of MS patients had normal memory or mild memory dysfunction, 30 per cent had moderate dysfunction, and 30 per cent had severe impairment. However, memory decline can also be related to anti-anxiety medication. It is not related to the degree of physical disability, disease duration and depression. One of the most frustrating cognitive deficits seen in MS is having a word on the tip of your tongue and not being able to remember it.

The first signs of cognitive impairment are often subtle. You may forget what you were about to say, fail to pass on certain information, have difficulty in finding the right words, or start to demonstrate poor judgement. It is often the family who becomes aware of these problems first. Cognitive dysfunction can interfere with your ability to fulfil your role at home and at work. Together with fatigue, it is a leading reason for taking early retirement in those with MS.

If you would like your cognitive function to be assessed, a trained health professional – either a neuropsychologist, speech/language pathologist or occupational therapist – should be able to offer you a series of tests from which your cognitive strengths and weaknesses can be determined. If some cognitive impairment is detected, you will be shown various strategies for coping.

Treatment of cognitive dysfunction

Because disease-modifying drugs (DMDs) have been proved to decrease the number of MS lesions in the central nervous system, it is assumed that cognitive deterioration will slow down over time. The drug donepezil hydrochloride (Aricept) has been developed to treat cognitive function directly, and slightly improves verbal memory in MS. Overall, as an important adjunct to DMDs, the best treatment for cognitive impairment is cognitive rehabilitation (as mentioned above), which teaches strategies from computer-mediated memory exercises to using memory aids such as notebooks and post-its, organization, computers, filing systems and so on.

Numerous studies are currently under way into finding the best means of dealing with cognitive changes.

Sexual dysfunction

Sex is an important part of any healthy relationship and it's distressing when there are problems. In MS, sexual dysfunction of some kind affects around 70 per cent of women and 90 per cent of men. Sexual arousal starts in the central nervous system when the brain uses the nerve pathways to send messages to the sexual organs. These nerve pathways are sometimes damaged in MS, and this affects different areas of sexual function. When fatigue and depression are also part of the equation, it's no wonder that distress can arise. MS can affect sexual experience in the following ways:

- Emotional issues – there may be anxiety, fear, feelings of inadequacy, etc.
- Failure to communicate effectively – your partner may not be aware of your difficulties.
- Incontinence – bladder control can be decreased during inter-course, which is embarrassing and off-putting.
- Pain can inhibit pleasure.
- Spasticity – when the legs are difficult to separate because of cramps or uncontrollable spasms, penetration can be difficult.
- Spasms – uncontrollable muscle movements can impede both desire and function.
- Concentration difficulties – it can be difficult to concentrate on what is happening.
- Self-image – the person feels 'sick' or 'ill', which can prevent arousal.
- Medications – the side-effects of certain drugs blunt sex drive.

Sexual performance
MS can have an effect on both men and women before and during sexual activity.

In women:

- Reduced sensation in the clitoral area of the vagina, or painfully heightened sensation.
- Vaginal dryness.
- Difficulty reaching orgasm.
- Loss of sex drive.

In men:

- Trouble achieving or keeping an erection.
- Decreased sensation in the penis.
- Difficulty achieving ejaculation.
- Loss of sex drive.

Treatment of sexual dysfunction

Speaking of your sexual problems to a medical professional is your first step towards finding a solution. (You have no need to feel shy about discussing sexual matters with your doctor – medics deal with such things all the time. It's an expected part of their job.)

For a man, there are several prescription medications available, including Viagra (sildenafil), injectable medications such as papaverine and phentolamine (Vasomax, Regitine and Z-Max) that boost blood flow to the penis, the MUSE system where a small suppository is inserted into the penis, as well as implants and inflatable devices.

For a woman, over-the-counter gels and liquid lubricants can relieve vaginal dryness. However, they must be used liberally to achieve the desired effect. It is not recommended to use Vaseline or other petroleum gels as they can lead to infection.

Reduced sensation and slow arousal can be overcome by using a vibrator together. Catheterization before intimacy can control the problem of incontinence during lovemaking. If you suffer from muscle spasms, you can use prescription medication to control them.

The psyche and sexual dysfunction in MS

Many psychological factors can impair sexual function in MS. For instance, some people find it difficult to reconcile the idea of being disabled with being sexually active. When combined with loss of self-esteem, demoralization, depression, anxiety, anger and the stress of living with a chronic illness, sexuality within a relationship can be severely challenged. The problem can be compounded when the man is the patient, and the woman the caregiver – he wants to continue taking the lead in their sex life, but it's not so easy. Furthermore, sexual intimacy is a way of expressing feelings of fulfilment within the relationship, yet the strain of coping with MS can emotionally distance the couple.

A study was conducted in Italy a few years ago in which the prevalence of sexual difficulties in people with MS, people with chronic illness and people without illness were compared, and all subjects were matched on sex and age. It was found that people with MS had the highest rates of sexual dysfunction (73.1 per cent) in contrast with the chronic illness group (39.2 per cent) and the healthy group (12.7 per cent). In women, problems with libido, lack of vaginal lubrication and orgasm were mainly reported. In men, the chief problem was erectile dysfunction. More work is clearly required to understand the sexual problems faced by people with MS.

Fortunately, there are ways and means to tackle most sexual difficulties. Once you have spoken to your doctor, you will be referred for counselling to a mental health professional or trained sexual therapist. Both psychological and physiological issues will be addressed.

Emotional issues

Unfortunately, there are profound emotional consequences to having MS. Adjusting to the diagnosis is far from easy, and a lack of knowledge about the disease only contributes to an already heavy load of anxiety. Some emotional changes are due to demyelination and damage to nerve fibres in the central nervous system. Many of the medications used in MS can also impact significantly on the emotions.

The emotional changes related to MS can include the following:

- Depression, or depressive symptoms of lesser severity. In a study of 40 people with MS, with the length of their diagnoses ranging from 1 year to 31 years, the majority of people gave evidence of hidden depression, with overt depression being the second most frequent response. Overt depression was shown to increase with the progression of functional limitations, while denial seemed to decrease.

- Grieving for the losses linked with the disease.
- Stress.
- Anxiety.
- Distress, particularly when faced with a difficult situation related to MS.
- The 'pseudobulbar affect' (PBA), also known as 'uncontrollable laughing and/or crying'.
- Emotional lability. Lability means liable to change, easily altered, and is present in MS when the person either starts laughing inappropriately or bursts into tears for no apparent reason. Mood swings can be caused by lability, as can inappropriate sexual behaviour such as sexual aggressiveness. However, in the above-mentioned study of 40 people with MS, only two displayed evidence of lability.
- Euphoria. Sufferers have often been characterized as euphoric in their emotional response to the disease – euphoric in this instance means having an unrealistic and inappropriately optimistic attitude towards the illness, or an abnormal sense of well-being. However, the above-mentioned study indicated that this is frequently a mask for underlying depression, and that people with MS experience a spectrum of feelings – depressed feelings at one end of the scale and euphoria at the other. The people in the study showed little evidence of elevated moods (euphoria), and it was hypothesized that any euphoria present in a person might be derived from the frequent remissions characteristic of the illness.
- General emotional instability, involving anger, frustration and irritability, all of which are connected to the process of adapting to a chronic disease.

Drugs called cholinesterase inhibitors have been shown to be of benefit to cognitive function and emotional distress. It is also thought that vocational programmes, where the person is given work of some kind, can be helpful too. In some areas, there are also therapeutic programmes for the person with MS and his or her family. These programmes can help the person affected to better understand and cope with cognitive weaknesses, such as concentration and problem solving. They also provide an excellent resource for families.

Speech problems

Difficulties with speech are fairly common in MS and there are several types of problem. The business of speaking is a highly complicated process, relying on the muscles being finely co-ordinated and controlled. In some people with weak 'speech' muscles, the problem is barely noticeable, but sadly, with others, the person clearly has difficulty making the right speech sounds and his or her voice sounds distorted. Speech problems are called 'dysarthria' and involve the tongue, lips, jaw and soft palate – the back part of the roof of the mouth.

Speech is controlled by many different areas within the central nervous system, so difficulties can depend on where lesions are located. Voice loudness and pitch may be hard to control – it may switch to high volume at inappropriate times, or be so low at other times that it is hard to decipher. Due to mal-coordination of the muscles that control the lips, tongue or soft palate, consonants may not sound quite right. In some people with MS, their speech sounds slurred; in others, they have 'scanning speech', in which they speak very slowly and pause after almost every syllable. In other people, their voice sounds very different from normal, becoming hoarse, nasal, harsh or pitched too high or too low. It can also sound shaky, due to tremor, or there may be long gaps between words.

Speech problems can be accompanied by tremor, head shaking and mal-coordination.

Communication

Changes in speech can make it difficult to communicate effectively, but may be less of a stumbling block to family, carers and close friends, for not only are you more relaxed with people you are familiar with, but also these people see you regularly enough to become accustomed to the way you speak.

It is when you are making a purchase from an unfamiliar shop, trying to explain a problem to the plumber, or being asked for your order in a restaurant that you can feel intensely self-conscious and frustrated – even foolish – as you struggle to speak. Meeting friends who haven't seen you in a while can also be difficult, especially if they have not been forewarned. The telephone is also a problematic area, especially for calls to people who don't know and understand you. It can be tempting to let others make your phone calls for you, or do the buying and ordering – but I would recommend that you keep trying. If the person to whom you are speaking grows impatient, it indicates that he or she has character flaws, while you are displaying only strength and determination.

If you have problems with your speech, you wouldn't be human if you didn't feel frustrated. Being unable to communicate easily can even make you feel left out or overlooked. However, people with MS seem to find an extraordinary inner strength, not to mention innovativeness, when they face such problems. For instance, with family, close friends and carers, you may develop a whole series of signals.

Speech and language therapy

Speech can be improved by a skilled speech and language therapist, so try to see a therapist as soon as you detect a speech problem. Each case is judged individually, and a plan of action will be tailored to your particular needs. A speech therapist will work with you on a one-to-one basis, building up a bond of empathy and trust. The therapy will aim to improve your breathing, enunciation and oral communication in general. Your homework will be a variety of exercises to perform in your own time.

Your doctor or neurologist can make the appropriate referral. It's most unlikely that you will lose your ability to speak altogether, but if it does happen, communication aid equipment is available. These range from alphabet cards to hand-held communicators that print out a tape. There are also computers that speak in response to eye blinks.

Problems with swallowing

Many people with speech problems also have difficulty in swallowing (dysphagia), for some of the nerves dealing with speech and swallowing are close companions in the central nervous system. However, not everyone with speech problems develops swallowing difficulties. They normally arise in a small percentage of people in the advanced stages of MS – but they are capable of arising at any time. The symptoms of a swallowing problem include the following:

- Coughing or choking when eating.
- Inhaling foods into the windpipe (trachea) instead of swallowing it down the gullet.
- The feeling that food is lodged in the throat.

Sadly, a person who frequently inhales food and drink causes it to be taken down into the windpipe and into the lungs, where abscesses then develop. Also, as a result of foreign bodies – in this case, food and drink – being present in the lungs, recurrent lung infections occur, which are known as pneumonia. When insufficient food and liquid reach the stomach, malnutrition and dehydration are a distinct possibility.

The person will normally experience unpleasant sensations when food and liquid are taken down the windpipe, so it is clear to that person what has happened. However, small amounts of food and liquid may be inhaled without the person being aware of it. This is called 'silent aspiration'.

Seeing your doctor

Your doctor will ask questions about the nature of your problem, after which a physical examination of your tongue and swallowing muscles will be carried out. Before a diagnosis can be given, it may be recommended that you have a test called a modified barium swallow, before which you will need to drink or eat a special 'contrast' substance in different consistencies – thin liquid, thick liquid and solid. As you do this, a machine will take pictures tracing the path of the substance. In this way, the exact location and manner of swallowing can be identified.

Treatment of swallowing problems

Swallowing problems are usually treated by a speech and language therapist. You will be encouraged to change your diet and the positioning of your head as you eat. You will also be shown a series of beneficial exercises or stimulation designed to improve swallowing. In the few very severe cases that fail to respond, a feeding tube may have to be inserted directly into the stomach to provide nutrition and fluids.

The following tips should make swallowing easier:

- As you eat, sit upright with your head tilted forward slightly at the neck.

- Eat slowly. Cut your food into small pieces and chew each one thoroughly. Don't eat more than half a teaspoonful of food at a time.
- While you eat, don't be distracted by the television or radio, and don't read, send a text or do a crossword puzzle.
- Remember to swallow often – maybe two or three times per bite of food.
- If food or liquid catches in your throat, cough gently or clear your throat and swallow again before taking a breath.
- Try to alternate a bite of food with a drink of liquid. If you need to use a straw to drink and find it difficult to draw the liquid right up the straw, shorten the straw.
- Ensure that the food you eat isn't too hot. The same goes for drinks.
- Make foods easier to swallow by changing their texture. Puree in a blender if necessary.
- Prepare pureed food in the shape of real food – the psychological impact is surprising.
- If soft foods make you cough, thicken them with cornflour. Instead of using thin soups, eat creamy soups. Drink the more 'gutsy' fruit juices, as well as Horlicks, Bovril and so on.
- Drink plenty of fluids. Every now and then, suck on an ice lolly or flavoured ice cube or drink home-made lemonade. These will increase the saliva in your mouth.
- Remain upright for at least three-quarters of an hour after finishing your meal.
- Crush your pills and mix them with pudding or jam. It might be best to ask your pharmacist whether it's all right to crush your particular pills. Speak to your doctor about this too. You might be prescribed liquid medications that are easier to get down.
- You may need to work with an otolaryngologist – a doctor specializing in ear, nose and throat disorders – to address your swallowing problems. Left untreated, swallowing problems can increase your risk of developing pneumonia, malnutrition, dehydration and other problems.

3

Diagnosis

If you suspect you have MS, it is important that you see your doctor as soon as possible. I realize it must be incredibly frightening to think you have MS, but for most people there are definite advantages to seeing their doctor in the early stages of the disease:

- Experts believe the disease is less likely to progress if you are having treatment.
- The earlier you start treatment, the quicker you will discover the drug that works best for you. There are many different drugs.

If your doctor thinks MS is a possibility, you are likely to be referred to a neurologist. Try to form a close relationship with both your doctor and neurologist, for if you do have MS, the type of relationship where you can speak openly of what you feel are intimate, embarrassing and distressing problems will be of benefit to you both. A good relationship with medical professionals helps you to feel supported and understood.

Seeing your doctor

To help your doctor to assess the situation, offer as much information as you can about any symptoms you have. Some details may be embarrassing – regarding bladder control and sexual function, for example – but they really should be mentioned. Your doctor's role is to calmly look at your symptoms, ask questions, then attempt to fit the pieces together. Some tips follow:

- In fear of being judged, don't be tempted to censor your descriptions of certain symptoms – that is, anxiety, depression, etc.
- Don't bombard – and therefore confuse – the doctor with your symptoms. Speak slowly and calmly and you'll be better understood.
- In deference to the doctor's lack of time, don't be tempted to describe only your main symptom(s), omitting those that may otherwise help the doctor to draw a clearer picture.

The diagnosis

Currently, there is no single test available to identify MS. Instead, several tests and procedures are required for diagnosis. The most recent diagnostic criteria were published in 1983 in the *Annals of Neurology* by Poser *et al.* Its main features are described below.

Medical history

Your doctor will need an overall picture of your health. Bear in mind that the huge variety of possible MS symptoms is astounding. Your symptoms may include numbness, weakness in a limb or visual disturbance of some kind, usually in the form of loss of visual sharpness, a blind spot, or loss of colour vision – all affecting one eye. On the other hand, your symptoms may be tingling, muscle tightness, poor sensation and so on. Less frequently, symptoms may be dizziness, unsteady gait, double vision, tremor or even sexual dysfunction.

It is important that you tell your doctor every single symptom you've experienced, not just the problems you think might be associated with MS. Also, don't just tell your doctor about your most recent problems. If you've had problems in the past, you must let the doctor know.

Nervous system function

You can expect your doctor to test your reflexes, balance, co-ordination and vision. There are specific ways your doctor can do this, such as using a small medical hammer to tap your knees and so judge the reflex.

Your doctor will also ask whether you have areas of numbness.

The diagnostic tests

If your doctor suspects you have MS, you will be sent for one or more of the following tests:

MRI scans

The widespread use of MRI (Magnetic Resonance Imaging) has recently transformed the diagnosis of MS. Indeed, MS-related lesions in the brain and spinal cord can be detected in over 90 per cent of suspected cases, making MRI far more successful where MS is concerned than even the CAT scan. Lesions fail to be detected in 5 per cent of MS patients.

The MRI scan produces very clear pictures of the human body without the use of X-rays. Instead, a large magnet, radio waves and a computer are used, making it very safe. MRI is even safe if you have surgical clips, sutures or staples, artificial joints, brain shunt tubes and cardiac valve replacements – except for the Starr-Edwards metallic ball or cage. It is even safe for people who have had other types of heart surgery.

You should tell your doctor, however, if you are pregnant, have a heart pacemaker, a cerebral aneurysm clip, implanted insulin pump, severe lung disease, gastric reflux, implanted spine stabilization rods, metal in the eye or eye socket, weigh more than 300 lbs (136 kg), or suffer from claustrophobia – the fear of confined spaces.

The scan takes between 40 and 80 minutes, during which time dozens of pictures may be taken. During the scanning you are likely to hear a muffled thumping sound, but you should experience no unusual sensations. All you need to do is lie on your back.

Evoked potential tests

Evoked potential tests are generally carried out when MS is suspected and a neurological examination alone – see 'nervous system function' above – does not provide sufficient evidence. The tests measure the time it takes for the nervous system to respond to certain stimuli. They also measure the size of the response.

The types of response induced are as follows:

- Stimulation of hearing by listening to a test tone through earphones.
- Stimulation of the arms and legs via an electrical pulse at the wrist or knee. This pulse is felt as a small electric shock.
- Stimulation of the eyes by looking at a test pattern. Around 80 per cent of people with MS have slow visual responses. This is therefore the most specific and reliable test for helping to diagnose MS.

Each type of response is recorded from the brainwaves through electrodes that are taped to the scalp. The location of the electrodes depends on whether the technician wants to test your hearing, limbs or vision.

Spinal tap

The spinal tap – also called a lumbar puncture – will only be carried out when MRI and evoked potential tests fail to produce a conclusive result. Spinal tap is a procedure that removes fluid from the spinal canal by means of a long thin needle inserted into the low back. When the fluid extracted reveals a large number of immuno-globulins (antibodies) or the breakdown products of myelin, the white jelly that protects the central nervous system nerve cells, MS is suspected. If MRI and evoked potential tests have also shown features of MS, it is likely that a diagnosis of MS will now be given.

Spinal tap is a safe procedure. However, a small number of people develop a headache afterwards, an even smaller number contract an infection and, occasionally, when a blood vessel has been pierced during the procedure, a 'bloody tap' will result, in which there is bleeding for a while. No treatment is required. If you develop a fever or any pain worsens, call your doctor immediately.

Making the diagnosis

Your neurologist will look closely at your test results, searching for signs of the disease in different parts of the central nervous system. Signs of at least two separate flare-ups of the disease will also be looked for – although this may be gained as much from questions as anything else.

Only when all the tests and your medical history are taken into account will a diagnosis of MS be given.

While tests are under way

It takes time to diagnose MS, and it's only natural that in the interim you will worry about the outcome. After all, from what your neighbour says about MS – her niece has it – that's what you have too! There will always be people who insist on diagnosing for you, often making a poor outlook appear a real probability. But such people are rarely knowledgeable enough on the subject to also tell you that there is good treatment for MS that can slow down the disease process.

Of course, if you don't have a neighbour, friend or relative who is keen to tell you what's wrong with you, your own mind is likely to be working overtime. If you are in that situation at the moment, undergoing tests or awaiting their results, remember that MS is by no means a death sentence – you are more likely to die of cancer or a road traffic accident. MS is not a wheelchair sentence, either. As stated earlier, three-quarters of people with MS don't ever need to use a wheelchair. Moreover, most manage to live productive, satisfying lives.

When you receive the diagnosis

I doubt there is one person with MS who doesn't have a clear memory of the doctor – usually a neurologist – who gave them their diagnosis. Memories of the strong feelings they experienced at the time – anger, confusion, frustration and so on – will stay with them for ever, for the diagnosis is a pivotal point in anyone's life. Even if you were expecting the diagnosis, the shock is just as intense, for how can you truly be prepared to be told you are suffering from a serious disease? I believe it's impossible.

When you are given the diagnosis in a casual manner, your shock is likely to be doubled. Fortunately, doctors nowadays are attempting to deliver the news in a more sensitive way, in the presence of a specialist MS nurse who is there to answer your questions and give you details of your nearest MS support group.

Even when the news is given with sympathy and optimism, it's common to feel angry with medical professionals. After all, it's the twenty-first century and doctors are carrying out miraculous procedures every day. Why is it then that they can't cure MS? Of course, part of your anger in the early days is likely to be your inability to understand what is happening to your body. In most cases the family tries hard to be supportive, yet at times they clearly need reassurance from you – that you are still the same person, that you won't become too ill, too cantankerous. Worst of all, the people you love seem to be looking at you differently, and you fear they are seeing only the disease and not the person beneath it.

How you react personally

Individuals react very differently to a diagnosis of serious illness. For some people, the trauma is more pronounced than for others. You might be the type of person who prefers to keep the news to yourself while you come to terms with it as much as you can, or you may want everyone to know so they can support you.

You may even be determined to keep your diagnosis a secret, feeling that apart from medical professionals, no one should know. There are numerous reasons you may feel this way, such as fearing being dismissed from your job, of worrying your family, of your partner leaving you, and so on. In the end, it is *your* life and you have a perfect right to tell who you wish – and *not* tell who you wish. However, if no one knows about your MS, you won't feel supported or understood. It's probably also important that you inform your employers to ensure you get treated fairly.

Seeing your neurologist

Prior to your first visit, make a note of all your symptoms, for it is easy to forget the details when you are anxious, along with any concerns and questions. 'What happens if I get a new symptom?' 'Could my child possibly develop MS?' or 'Will a future pregnancy worsen my symptoms?'

Ideally, ask about a 'care plan', inclusive of nutrition, food supplements, exercise and physical and occupational therapy. If your neurologist omits to discuss a plan of action, bring up the subject yourself, either at this appointment or the next.

MS facts

You have probably seen people with MS whose hands shake a lot as they try to pay for something, who are unable to walk without the aid of a stick, or who are so exhausted all the time they need to use a wheelchair. But this is only a brief peek at the whole MS story. What you may not be aware of are the following important points:

- It is possible to stay in the relapsing-remitting stage of MS for many years – even a lifetime – particularly if you take measures to help yourself. These measures include eliminating 'reactive' foods from your diet, staying as stress-free as possible, using complementary therapies, pacing yourself, learning to say 'no' and so on.
- Accepting drug-therapy early on in the disease gives you a fighting chance of minimizing any later disability.

- There are several disease-modifying drugs available and, if you work with your doctor or neurologist, you should find the drug that works best for you – and that will make all the difference to your prognosis. If you are experiencing side-effects, or are having more relapses than expected, talk to your neurologist. He or she may be able to prescribe a more appropriate medication.
- A great deal of research into the causes and treatment of MS is currently under way. Headway is being made all the time.

4

Treatment options

For many years, doctors could do little to treat MS. They were able to prescribe drugs to ease some of the symptoms, but nothing could change the course of the disease. We still don't have a cure for MS, but we do now have drugs that are capable of modifying the disease process in a large number of people.

When evaluating new treatments for MS, one of the greatest problems faced by researchers is the variability of the disease. Hence, a treatment that shows positive results in one person may not be in the slightest bit effective in another. I'm pleased to report, however, that the number of clinical trials for new MS treatments has gained pace in recent years, and that there are currently a great many important drug trials under way.

These are the two therapeutic courses of action in the treatment of MS:

- The use of drugs that can temper the disease, either slowing it down or stopping it.
- The use of drugs and other therapies that can ease or reduce specific symptoms, such as during a relapse.

Disease-modifying drugs

In MS, the reality of the diagnosis is generally not fully absorbed before you are being asked to decide whether you want to take drugs for specific symptoms or whether you wish to use drugs that can modify the course of the disease (known as DMDs – disease-modifying drugs). In considering DMDs, your neurologist and MS nurse will be only too happy to discuss with you the issues surrounding these drugs.

Studies have shown that nerves can be damaged very early on in MS (Weiner, 2004). Many neurologists believe, therefore, that DMD treatment should begin as soon as possible and they routinely prescribe these drugs at diagnosis. However, others question whether people should be introduced so early to a routine of injecting drugs. Moreover, the variable nature of MS means that some people can stay well without treatment for many years after diagnosis. The drugs sometimes carry side-effects, too – some of them serious. As yet, it is not known for sure whether they have long-term benefits.

In the end, whether you start using DMDs straightaway or leave it a while is your decision. However, the following should be considered before you make your choice:

For DMDs:

- Experts advise that DMDs are most effective when started very soon after the diagnosis, particularly if the disease is showing rapid advancement at an early stage.
- The same experts agree that DMDs can either slow down or stop the course of the disease.
- MRI scans have revealed a reduction in lesions in many people who take DMDs.
- As a result of the formation of fewer lesions, relapses tend to be of a shorter duration and less severe. Indeed, in clinical trials over a two-year period, DMDs decreased relapse rate by about 30 per cent. In other trials, DMDs were shown to reduce the severity of relapses.
- Because fewer lesions develop, the accumulation of disabilities seems to slow down.
- DMDs are currently the best defence available.
- Drugs for specific symptoms invariably carry long-term side-effects.

Against DMDs:

- Around 20 per cent of people with MS do well with no drug intervention at all (note that this is a relatively small percentage, however).
- Some people experience no benefit at all from DMDs.
- DMDs have been in use for five to ten years, but there is little data on how effective they are over that length of time.
- DMDs are believed to provide only a 30 per cent reduction in the onset of relapses.

- DMDs can cause depression, as well as blood and liver abnormalities. Therefore regular blood tests are mandatory.
- DMDs have to be administered by injection.
- There can be reddening, hardening or painful bruising at the injection site.
- Injections can cause flu-like symptoms at first.
- Some people are unable to commit themselves to the process of regular injections on a long-term basis.
- The long-term side-effects of DMDs are, as yet, not known.

Beta interferon

Beta interferon – an approved DMD – has been developed for the treatment of people with the relapsing-remitting form of MS. Approximately 40 per cent of patients have this type of MS, and it is characterized by acute relapses alternating with complete or partial recovery.

The discovery of beta interferon

Because MS researchers believe that an environmental agent or infection may trigger the disease in certain people, the possibility was raised that gamma interferon, one of the body's natural weapons against viruses, might help to fight the disease. In 1984, researchers administered gamma interferon to MS patients, but unfortunately their symptoms worsened considerably. This caused researchers to wonder whether gamma interferon itself might be directly involved in MS. Consequently, they monitored gamma interferon levels in MS patients and found that the levels shot up just before and during relapses.

This discovery raised the suggestion that beta interferon, which impedes the action of gamma interferon, could be a beneficial treatment of MS. Using cultured cells from MS patients, researchers found that beta interferon slowed down the growth of immune system cells – those that cause inflammation in the central nervous system. It was also discovered that beta interferon halts the production of the compounds that destroy myelin and correct a deficiency in T-cells, the white blood cells that are part of the immune system.

The patients prescribed beta interferon were soon experiencing fewer, less severe attacks of MS and fewer hospitalizations. Notably, those taking high doses of beta interferon were shown on MRI scans to have fewer brain lesions than patients taking lower doses or a placebo.

In the UK, there are two licensed forms of interferon medication available. They are beta interferon 1a (two types: Avonex and Rebif) and beta interferon 1b (Betaferon). These are all treatments for relapsing-remitting MS. Betaferon and Rebif can also be useful for treating people with progressive MS who experience relapses. Unfortunately, beta interferon is not able to help people who are already severely disabled – that is, no longer able to walk.

Scientists are now attempting to fully demystify the components of myelin, for it is one or more of these that trigger the immune system reaction. When all the components are known, they expect to develop better treatments and, eventually, a cure.

The side-effects of beta interferon

Beta interferon must be injected into a muscle, which can be difficult for some people. The drug frequently produces flu-like side-effects and inflammation at the injection site – however, these effects normally subside after a few months. The drug is also capable of causing depression, which may be severe.

Copaxone

There is now a synthetic form of DMD, called glatiramer acetate (Copaxone). This drug is a myelin basic protein designed to encourage the immune system to accept rather than attack the protective myelin. Copaxone is used to treat the relapsing-remitting form of MS.

Choosing the right DMD

In selecting the most suitable DMD for your needs, you would be advised to consider which type is best for the phase of MS you are currently experiencing. For instance, Avonex, Rebif and Betaferon can all be used in the treatment of relapsing-remitting MS, while

Betaferon and Rebif can be used in the treatment of progressive MS, where relapses still occur. Sadly, when MS is purely progressive, with no relapses, DMDs are generally ineffective. The criterion for the use of beta interferon, for people with relapsing-remitting MS, is given below.

You should also decide whether or not you can commit to regular injections for the foreseeable future. If you think you can, consider which cycle of injections will fit best into your lifestyle (see below).

Administration of DMDs

Betaferon, Rebif and Copaxone must be injected beneath the skin – Betaferon every other day, Rebif three times a week, and Copaxone daily. Avonex must be injected into muscle once a week. Betaferon needs mixing before use, but the other DMDs come ready to inject. Of course, self-injection is a tricky subject in itself, and not all people are able to do it. Before announcing that you just *can't* do it, look at the website www.msdecisions.org.uk where there is a great deal of information on every aspect of MS. There are also video clips showing people injecting in the correct way.

You can also ask your MS support nurse to help you to develop a good injection technique. As well as showing you how to inject, the nurse will encourage you to carry out the procedure in a relaxed, unrushed atmosphere, and to make it a normal part of your routine. If you think you'll need support with the process of giving injections, this must be discussed with your partner, a family member, friend, or your practice nurse. Unfortunately, oral forms of DMDs have proved ineffective.

The following pointers may help (Frohman *et al.*, 2004):

- Let the medication stand at room temperature before use.
- Ensure your environment is comfortable and relaxed, a place where you will not be disturbed.
- Wash your hands thoroughly.
- Apply an ice-pack to the area of skin to be injected. This should reduce any adverse skin reactions.
- Clean the area of skin to be injected.
- Don't discharge any liquid medication on to the outside of the needle before injecting.

- Use a different injection site each time, on a rotation system.
- Use an area where there is plenty of body fat.
- Try to make the injections a part of your normal routine.
- If you have any problems at all once you have begun injecting, go to your MS support nurse.

Auto-inject devices are now available, which make the injection easier. All DMDs must be stored in a cool place – preferably the fridge.

The criteria for use of beta interferon for people with relapsing-remitting MS (RR-MS)

In 2001, the Association of British Neurologists (ABN) issued guidelines for the use of beta interferons and glatiramer acetate (Copaxone) in MS. They should, the ABN said, be used only by people who fit into *all* of the following categories:

- If you are able to walk more than 100 metres without assistance, or if you can walk at least 10 metres, with or without assistance.
- If you have had two or more clinically significant relapses in the last two years.
- If you are 18 or over.
- If there are no contraindications (reasons that the drugs should not be taken, such as pregnancy or breastfeeding).

The criteria for the use of beta interferon for people with secondary-progressive MS (SP-MS)

In trials of people with secondary-progressive MS – where their MS began with the relapsing-remitting pattern and evolved into the progressive pattern – a 30 per cent reduction in relapse rate was observed as a result of taking beta interferon. The trial included people who were more disabled, but who could walk at least 10 metres without assistance.

According to ABN guidelines, beta interferon should be used only by people who fit into all of the following categories:

- If you are able to walk at least 10 metres with or without assistance.

- If you have experienced two or more disabling relapses in the last two years.
- If there is minimal increase in disability due to slow progression (not relapses) over the last two years.
- You should be 18 or over.
- There should be no contraindications.

The criteria for use of Copaxone (glatiramer acetate)

According to ABN guidelines, Copaxone should be used only by people who fit into all of the following categories:

- If you have relapsing-remitting MS. This treatment is not effective for other types of MS.
- If you are able to walk at least 100 metres without assistance.
- If you have experienced two or more clinically significant relapses in the last two years.
- If you are 18 or over.
- If there are no contraindications.

Stopping DMD treatment

According to the Association of British Neurologists, treatment should be stopped in the following circumstances:

- If you want to start trying for a baby. (In this instance, treatment should be stopped three months beforehand.)
- If you feel the treatment has not worked, or has stopped working.
- If the side-effects are unmanageable.
- If a treatment becomes available that is more suited to you.
- If you have experienced two severe relapses, as defined by your neurologist, over a 12-month period. If you are used to having more than two relapses, you may still be showing an improvement with the drug.
- If there is an obvious increase in disability over six months.
- If you experience one relapse that lasts for over six months, during which time there is increased disability.
- If you lose the ability to walk, even with assistance, for a period of six months.

Comparisons

As there have been no long-term studies of DMDs, it is not easy to compare one drug with another. However, they are believed to be equally effective.

Side-effects of DMDs

Until researchers come up with effective oral medication for MS, treatment in the form of DMDs must be administered by injection. In around 50 per cent of cases, DMD injections can cause reddening, hardening or painful bruising at the injection site.

After using beta interferon (Avonex, Rebif and Betaferon), approximately 50 per cent of people with MS experience periods of flu-like symptoms, such as muscle aches, fever, chills and headache, particularly after the first injection. Such symptoms are usually worse in the first three months of treatment, reducing over time. Taking ibuprofen (Advil, Motrin) or paracetamol (Panadol, Tylenol) will ease the symptoms. The Association of British Neurologists recommends injecting before bedtime so you sleep through the worst of the flu-like symptoms.

People taking beta interferon should have regular blood tests to check liver function and blood cell count. On rare occasions, this type of DMD can cause blood abnormalities such as mild anaemia, a reduction in white blood cell count, and changes in menstruation. Liver abnormalities can also occur.

The side-effects of Copaxone can include short-term chest tightness or pain, accompanied by sweating, flushing, anxiety, palpitations and a perceived difficulty in breathing. This occurs directly after an injection and can last between 30 seconds and 30 minutes. These symptoms may occur after a first dose, after several months, or not at all. No permanent or serious harm has been caused by these symptoms. With all DMDs, the side-effects in some people are serious enough to make them want to stop treatment. Your doctor or neurologist will speak to you about changing to another treatment, but whether you do so is your decision in the end.

In some people, beta interferons can provoke an immune response, where the immune system makes antibodies that block or 'neutralize' the action of the drug. This causes the drug to work less efficiently, particularly where relapses are concerned. However, an immune response will not cause the disease to worsen on a long-term basis. There is currently a great deal of research going on into the role of neutralizing antibodies.

Although DMDs have been in use for ten years to date, their effectiveness over five or ten years has been measured in very few studies. However, a ten-year NHS monitoring programme is currently under way. In addition, more DMDs are being developed by researchers. They are also evaluating blends of new and existing drugs for people who fail to respond to a single drug treatment.

Other disease-modifying drugs

Other DMDs used for treating MS are as follows:

Corticosteroids

Corticosteroids are natural hormones produced by the adrenal glands at times of stress. Synthetic versions of the hormone have been used for controlling MS since the 1950s, and are still the standard treatment for acute flare-ups. Because they suppress the immune system, reduce inflammation and are thought to prevent the leakage of harmful blood cells into the central nervous system, they can take the edge off a bad relapse. However, they can't stop the relapse or determine the outcome.

'Corticosteroids' is the blanket term for drugs such as methylprednisolone (Solu-Medrol) and dexamethasone (Decadron). Specialists believe that, during a severe relapse, a three- to five-day course of high-dose intravenous corticosteroids is the best way to reduce symptoms. Unfortunately, not all neurologists are willing to prescribe corticosteroids for relapses.

This type of drug should always be taken under medical supervision. Possible side-effects include water retention, stomach irritation, mood swings, insomnia and raised blood sugar levels. In most people, there are no adverse reactions, however.

Antegren

An ongoing two-year trial into the effects of this new drug has shown that, over a period of six months, people with relapsing-remitting MS develop fewer lesions than people not taking the drug (Miller *et al.*, 2003). The same people displayed a decreased number of relapses during that period too.

If the licence for use of this drug is approved, it will be administered by monthly infusion into a vein. Antegren works by interfering with the movement of potentially damaging immune cells, preventing them from passing into the central nervous system. A previous trial showed that the drug was well tolerated.

Campath 1H

This drug is also being tested before a licence can be given. It has been shown already to reduce relapse symptoms, but relatively serious side-effects emerged in the study subjects. Campath 1H is now undergoing a three-year trial.

Mitoxantrone (Novantrone)

Approved in the USA and licensed in the UK for treating secondary-progressive MS and deteriorating relapsing-remitting MS, mitoxantrone (brand name Novantrone) was first developed as an anti-cancer agent and acts like chemotherapy to increase immune cells when an invading organism is present. This drug, therefore, has the potential to be far more harmful than other MS treatment agents. However, in the UK, some people with aggressive relapsing-remitting MS are now being given this drug, and it would appear that the relief experienced outstrips any concern over harmful effects. Nevertheless, treatment courses are limited to between six months and two years.

Intravenous immunoglobulin (IVIg)

IVIg therapy is made up of non-specific human antibodies and must be injected or infused into a vein. MRI scans have suggested that IVIg lessens MS activity, and small-scale studies have indicated that it can decrease the number of relapses in some people. The therapy is sometimes used as a back-up to other DMDs. However, it is known to have no effect on secondary-progressive MS (Fazekas *et al.*, 1997).

Azathioprine (Imuran)

This drug (brand name Imuran) is used to treat diseases of immune system dysfunction. It works by impeding the rapid increase of white blood cells – the immune system. Its high risk of serious side-effects means it is rarely used to treat MS.

The risk-sharing scheme

It is now possible to be prescribed DMDs on the NHS, by means of what is known as the 'risk-sharing scheme'. Under the scheme, a person with MS who is given this type of drug will be observed for up to ten years, to monitor the effectiveness. DMDs are very expensive, therefore the Department of Health and the drug companies involved have agreed to share the cost until the result of the programme is known. If the outcome of treatment is disappointing and not as advocated by the drug companies, the NHS will pay less for DMDs.

Once a year, the NHS will assess people who have been given the drugs. The results will then be compared with the natural disease progression without DMD intervention. The long-term effects of DMDs will be discovered by this process.

Neurologists at MS assessment centres can prescribe DMDs, provided that you fit the ABN criteria for diagnosis of the disease. If you are interested in taking part in the scheme, speak to your doctor, MS nurse or neurologist with a view to them making a referral to a neurologist at one of the assessment centres. (Different areas of the UK have different referral procedures.) There are currently around 70 assessment centres throughout the UK.

Future treatments

Without DMDs, an acceleration in the loss of nerve fibres occurs, and drugs that alter immune system function are of little use once the loss reaches a certain point, generally when relapsing-remitting MS becomes progressive MS. Ideally, drugs that protect the nerve fibres and reduce immune attack need to be given to stop the progression of MS. Researchers are working on such drugs, which are termed 'neuroprotective'.

Symptomatic treatments

Because MS affects multiple areas of the central nervous system, a diverse array of symptoms can result. Early symptoms can be short-lived, but recovery is not always complete. Over time, the majority of people with MS develop an increasing range of relapse symptoms, with progressive worsening of their overall condition.

This section gives a brief outline of the treatments available for individual symptoms. They are all prescription medications and your doctor will discuss with you the appropriate ones in more detail.

Muscle spasticity

Stiffness and muscle spasms (known as spasticity) are common in MS. Recommended treatments include the following:

- Baclofen (Lioresal) – a muscle relaxant. The side-effects can include dizziness, drowsiness, fatigue and weakness.
- Diazepam (Valium) – a muscle relaxant. The side-effects can include drowsiness, dizziness and ataxia (i.e. loss of full control of body movements).
- Dantrolene (Dantrium) – a muscle relaxant. Possible side-effects include dizziness, weakness and diarrhoea.

Pain

The recommended treatment for the pain of MS includes the following:

- Amitriptyline (Elavil) – for the pain of muscle stiffness, spasms and so on. The possible side-effects include dry mouth, fatigue, confusion and urinary retention.
- Imipramine (Tofranil) – for the pain of muscle stiffness, spasms and so on. The side-effects can include dry mouth, dizziness, drowsiness, nausea and weight gain.
- Co-codamol 30/500 (Tylex) – an analgesic comprising 500 mg paracetamol and 30 mg codeine phosphate. Used for severe pain. The possible side-effects include dry mouth, nausea or blurred vision.
- Gabapentin (Neurontin) – for neuropathic (nerve) pain. The side-effects can include dizziness, fatigue, ataxia and involuntary eye movements (nystagmus).
- Pregabalin (Lyrica) – for neuropathic (nerve) pain. The side-effects for this newer treatment can include dizziness, fatigue and weight gain.

Fatigue

Fatigue can be one of the most disabling symptoms of MS and cannot as yet be treated effectively. However, the following medications can take the edge off the problem:

- Fluoxetine (Prozac) – an antidepressant. The side-effects can include anxiety, dizziness and anorexia.
- Methylphenidate (Ritalin) – a stimulant. The side-effects can include insomnia, seizures, liver dysfunction and anorexia.
- Amantidine (Symadine and Symmetrel) – an antiviral medication. Possible side-effects include nausea, dizziness and insomnia.

Bladder problems

Bladder problems in MS can be treated by the following bladder strengtheners:

- Oxybutynin (Ditropan XL/Detrol LA/Oxytrol patch) – side-effects can include dry mouth, drowsiness and urinary retention. A failure of the bladder to empty must be treated by catheterization.
- Propantheline (Probanthine) – side-effects can include dry mouth, drowsiness and urinary retention.
- Tolterodine (Detrol) – side-effects can include mild dry mouth and drowsiness.
- Imipramine (Tofranil) – side-effects can include dry mouth, fatigue, confusion and urinary retention.

Constipation

Constipation is a common problem in MS. Although natural treatments are recommended for this problem, drug therapy can include the following:

- Colchicine (Colbenemid) – an antimitotic. The side-effects can include short-lived abdominal pain, nausea and vomiting.

5

Further help

In addition to drug therapy, there is a great deal of help available for people with MS. For instance, physiotherapy can help, and home exercise is also essential to managing the condition, as an active person is less likely to develop bladder and bowel problems, osteoporosis, permanent muscle contractions, ulcerations of the skin, or abnormal blood clotting. Before you get started, however, it is advisable that you ask your doctor what form of physical activity he or she would recommend.

Exercise suggestions

Because regular exercise is of enormous benefit in MS, here are some exercise suggestions:

- An exercise routine should be designed to stimulate the muscles. However, the muscles should not be overloaded and overheated as this can temporarily block nerve conduction. Your doctor or physiotherapist may be able to give you an appropriate exercise sheet. If not, there are dozens of books in the library devoted to exercise. Try to put together your own regime, remembering to avoid heavy weights and not to make your movements fast and aggressive. Some people with MS can tolerate aerobic exercise, but some cannot. If you can, incorporate this into your regime.
- Muscle spasticity can be reduced by stretching and doing range-of-motion exercises. These, too, can be found in exercise instruction books and should be included in your routine.
- Exercising in water is particularly beneficial in MS. Water supports your body as you exercise, removing the shock factor and conditioning your muscles with the minimum of discomfort (see 'Aquatic exercise' below).

Cooling methods

When the body is overheated, nerves that are stripped of their myelin function less efficiently. This is why some MS symptoms worsen when you feel hot. As well as exercise, a steamy bathroom will create this effect for some people, and a hot day will do the same for others. Fortunately, this effect is temporary and once a normal body temperature is regained, the symptoms subside.

If you are unable to tolerate heat, the following measures may help to keep your body from overheating:

- Use air-conditioning in hot weather. Often a simple desk fan will do the trick.
- Don't set the thermostat too high on the central heating in winter.
- Avoid swimming in a heated pool.
- Take a cooling shower after exercise or other physical activity.
- If possible, wear the type of helmet that uses cold liquid to cool your head and neck, and therefore lower your core body temperature. This will reduce MS symptoms not only when you are exercising, but also when you are doing the ironing, washing the car and so on.

Physiotherapy

In a 2001 survey of people with MS, participants reported that physiotherapy is an important part of their treatment regime. There is even scientific research showing that physiotherapy is beneficial in MS. A 1996 study of people with mild to moderate disability from MS, carried out by Jack Petajan, showed that regular aerobic exercise, vigorous enough to raise the pulse and respiration rate, increased fitness, arm and leg strength and workout capacity. The participants also reported decreased depression, fatigue and anger, and they had improved bowel and bladder control.

A physiotherapist will explain what is happening within your body and provide you with the tools to work on your particular problems. For example, you may unconsciously walk with a lopsided gait, drag a leg or have poor general posture – a lot of people with MS do. If this is the case, your physiotherapist will show you how to correct your posture and so improve your muscle tone and joint mobility, and will also help you to correct any balance and co-ordination problems. Where bladder and bowel problems are concerned, pelvic floor physiotherapy can be very useful. It may be best to take a cooling shower after exercise and physiotherapy to counter overheated muscles.

Ideally, physiotherapy should be started as early as possible, before the disease can inflict too much damage. Future complications can then either be reduced or avoided. You may find you are given a concentrated exercise regime to begin with, comprising stretching, strengthening, mobility and aerobic exercise. These exercises will help to counter fatigue, build up your strength, and help you to stay supple. It is important to note that people who are severely disabled through MS can still benefit from physiotherapy. In this instance, exercise may mostly comprise another person moving your limbs for you, perhaps with the assistance of painkillers or muscle relaxants.

If you can discipline yourself to carry out your prescribed exercise regime on a regular basis, you will not only improve strength and mobility in all areas of your body, you will also be helping yourself to maintain an optimistic outlook on life. You are doing something positive for yourself that is making a difference, and that knowledge makes you feel good.

Aquatic exercise

A water temperature of between 83 and 85 degrees Fahrenheit provides the very best exercise conditions for a person with MS. Water reduces the effects of gravity and the buoyancy or weightlessness helps a person with weakened limbs to attain a greater range of motion. Water that is chest high can provide support, enabling you to stand and maintain balance with less effort than on land. The pressure of the water also causes your chest to expand, encouraging deeper breathing and increasing oxygen intake.

Rather than exercising alone, many people prefer to join an aqua aerobics class. Most public swimming pools run aqua aerobic sessions, some of which are graded according to ability. As with all exercises, aqua aerobics are only truly beneficial when performed on a regular basis, so try to take up something that's easy to continue.

Muscle strengthening exercise is generally possible in water, where it may not be possible on land for some people with MS. For strengthening in water, there are now commercially available devices that can increase water resistance. Specific techniques can also be performed in water to address particular mobility problems.

Exercising in water helps to prevent the body from overheating, too.

Occupational therapy

Occupational therapy can provide a wide range of practical help at home, at work or in your leisure time. By learning alternative ways to complete different tasks, or with the introduction of specific equipment, a person with MS can perform everyday activities with greater ease and improve any limitations.

Occupational therapy equipment can help with the following:

- Looking after yourself. There are adaptations for bathing, showering and toilet use, dressing aids, grooming aids, and eating and dinnerware adaptations.
- Functioning well – at home, work, or in a place of learning. Useful equipment can include cooking and cleaning adaptations, handwriting aids, and keyboard and telephone modifications.
- Getting around. Occupational therapy can provide you with a wheelchair. It doesn't matter that you may only use it once a month when you feel tired, or when you're experiencing your annual relapse. On such occasions it will improve your ability to function. You may also be provided with a stick if you need one.
- Having fun. An occupational therapist can help you to enjoy hobbies and find new ways to get pleasure out of life. Leisure skill equipment can be provided.

Other help provided by occupational therapy includes the following:

- Information and advice on modifying your home for wheelchair use and so on.
- An evaluation on possible adaptations to your car, so you can continue or resume driving. Motability is a registered UK charity which enables disabled people to use the Higher Rate Mobility Component of their Disability Living Allowance to lease or buy a car or buy a powered wheelchair or scooter. Alternatively,

occupational therapy may provide information about modifying your present vehicle. See the 'Useful addresses' section (pages 122–7).

6

Pregnancy in MS

Because MS is more common in women of childbearing age than in any other group, pregnancy is an obvious issue and women naturally have many questions on the subject. They include:

- Is it responsible to get pregnant when I have MS?
- Will my MS worsen if I get pregnant?
- Would the pregnancy be difficult because of MS?
- Would the child be at risk of developing MS?

Is it wise to get pregnant when you have MS?

Whether or not you decide to get pregnant is entirely up to you. There are many factors to consider. For a start, you should take into account the unpredictable nature of MS and how this might impact on a growing child. Children demand time, patience and a great deal of energy. You need to know, therefore, that there is plenty of practical support on hand before you even think of getting pregnant. More emotional factors, such as how badly you want a child and the fact that children make you feel fulfilled, will obviously be part of the equation too.

Most doctors advise not taking medications, or changing to safer ones, for three to six months prior to conception. It is important you discuss this with your doctor. Some MS drugs are unsafe during pregnancy and breastfeeding, and you will have to manage without them – a further consideration.

The risk to the child

MS is not directly inherited, but genetic factors are thought to play a role in a small number of people. However, MS does not cause miscarriage or infertility, and it is not considered a medical risk to the foetus or newborn. The chances of passing on MS to your child are only 1–5 per cent, depending on the sex of the child and which parent has the disease. The probability is highest if it is the mother who has MS and if the baby is a girl. MS can also arise in 0.3 per cent of cases where the mother is disease-free and there is no indication of the disease in the family.

Does MS worsen with pregnancy?

For most women, the number and severity of MS relapses decrease during pregnancy, especially during the last few months. At this time, the disease can be as much as 70 per cent improved from pre-pregnancy. This is largely due to the fact that pregnancy mildly suppresses the immune system to protect the unborn child. Levels of natural corticosteroids are higher in pregnant women than non-pregnant women, which also makes a difference.

Unfortunately, there's a 20–40 per cent chance of relapses occurring in the postpartum period – that is, during the first 3–6 months after the birth. However, postpartum relapses don't appear to contribute to increased long-term disability. Indeed, studies have shown that of women with MS who gave birth, no increased disability as a result of pregnancy was found in the long term.

In later pregnancy, when your centre of gravity shifts, walking may be difficult – especially if you had gait problems beforehand. You may need to use a stick or even a wheelchair for a short time, and other devices may need to be employed. If you have pre-existing bladder and bowel problems, they may worsen in pregnancy. Fatigue may also be a prominent factor.

The right time to get pregnant

It is wise to plan the timing of your pregnancy. Conceiving during a remission is recommended as it gives yourself and the baby the best possible start. If you have experienced a severe relapse, waiting for up to two years before getting pregnant can give you a fighting chance of enjoying the pregnancy. Being in a stable condition prior to conception means you are less likely to experience a relapse after the birth.

Pregnancy and labour

In the second half of your pregnancy you may not be as protected from MS symptoms as you are in the first half, but you should experience fewer relapses. The symptoms you will be vulnerable to include fatigue, constipation and urinary tract infections, which are already symptoms of MS. An obstetrician may suggest that you use a stool softener to counter constipation, and that you give regular urine samples for analysis to detect possible infections.

You are as likely as a healthy woman to either bloom in pregnancy, or feel thoroughly unwell. As you near full term and become heavier and more ungainly, you may find you are less steady on your feet. It's a good idea, before you reach this stage, to install grab rails in your house, especially in the bathroom. Women with pronounced numbness or paralysis are likely to be closely monitored during the ninth month in case they are unable to detect the onset of contractions. In such women, labour may need to be induced when the cervix begins to open.

When a woman with MS is in labour, she is treated in much the same way as a healthy woman. The type of pain relief given may depend on the particular beliefs of your obstetrician. Epidural anaesthesia and general anaesthesia are tolerated well by women with MS. Pethidine – a synthetic version of morphine – may also be given. This drug is an antispasmodic that helps you to relax.

Women with MS can anticipate a normal delivery, and afterwards any weakness or spasms in the legs will be watched for and treated by the midwife or obstetrician.

Can medications be taken during pregnancy?

Because it would be unethical to carry out trials into the effects of medications on pregnancy, there is little data available about the risk to a foetus. Even so, of the existing reports, none has ever laid a claim to being completely risk-free. Most prospective MS mothers tend to err on the side of caution, taking no drugs at all during the first three months of pregnancy, when the child's organs are developing. In the event of a relapse in the first three months of pregnancy, this cannot be treated with high dose steroids until later on. If you are not planning to breastfeed, disease-modifying drugs can be restarted straight after delivery.

If you unknowingly become pregnant while taking medication – including disease-modifying drugs, and drugs for depression, spasticity, pain, fatigue, and bladder and bowel problems – you would be best advised to come off them straightaway, under the supervision of your doctor or neurologist. It is important to give your baby the best chance of developing properly. For pain and spasticity occurring during pregnancy and breastfeeding, take advantage of natural methods such as heat pads, ice packs, wheat bags, massage and so on. Stretching exercises, Pilates, yoga, aqua exercise and swimming can also be helpful.

After the birth

An ongoing trial is examining whether intravenous immunoglobulin therapy (IVIg), administered at the time of delivery to 100 women with MS (10 g or 60 g), followed by monthly IVIg (10 g) for six months, can prevent postpartum relapses. The chances of a relapse are always raised after the birth in MS. You should therefore try to take good care of yourself, getting enough rest and attempting to avoid stress, infections, fevers and anaemia. If you start to feel very tired, enlist help so you can sleep and relax more. If you are feeling particularly anxious and stressed, try to work out what exactly is causing it and aim to make your world calmer and more relaxed.

Research suggests that the chance of a relapse occurring after the birth increases in almost 50 per cent of cases. If you've experienced relapses in the past, the chances of one presenting itself following the birth are so much greater. Remember, however, that any worsening of symptoms is likely to be temporary. Within a year of giving birth, you should have reverted to your pre-pregnant condition.

Breastfeeding

Whether or not you breastfeed your baby is down to personal choice and whether you feel you can go without many of your normal drugs. Women who are taking the disease-modifying drugs Avonex, Betaferon, Rebif, Copaxone or Novantrone are not recommended to do so during breastfeeding as the drug can be excreted in the milk. If you use benzodiazepines such as diazepam (Valium), it is advised that you stop for the duration of breastfeeding. The use of prednisone, on the other hand, should be carefully monitored. On the other hand, you may prefer to bottle-feed and continue taking your disease-modifying drugs and other medications.

In most cases a woman with MS will successfully breastfeed her baby, if that's what she wants. If you are pregnant, it is recommended that you discuss breastfeeding with your obstetrician, paediatrician and neurologist before you decide whether to go ahead. Studies have shown no raised risk of relapse as a result of breastfeeding. However, there is some evidence of a small risk to the child by *not* breastfeeding, with studies indicating that infants fed only on cows' milk can have a higher than normal risk of developing MS in adulthood. Some milk proteins appear to carry a higher risk than others, but at present there's no way the average woman can tell them apart. Breast milk, on the other hand, contains factors that may help to regulate the immune response.

Breastfeeding can be very tiring for some mothers, and they can feel anxious about whether the child is getting enough milk. If you can't find ways of resting more and calming your anxieties, you may wish to change to bottle-feeding.

Bringing up your child

Being a new mother makes all women feel insecure. Add MS to the equation and the feeling of insecurity is multiplied a thousandfold. Among other things you worry that the fatigue, relapses and variety of other symptoms will make you an inadequate mother. The fact is, though, that it is the bond between the child and yourself, the closeness you share, the affection you show and the morals you teach, that make you a good mother.

If you find yourself worrying about the ironing, the cleaning, the unwashed kitchen floor – don't. So long as you keep kitchen work surfaces clean and sterilize your baby's bottles, there's no need to worry about the creased clothes, the dust, the dirty floor. Of course, you need things like clean clothes and nutritious foods, so rope in all those who promised their help. A recent MS survey showed that it was those women who were brave enough to ask for help who managed motherhood the best, and who had the most contented children. It's good, too, for your child to be used to having other people around. Not only does it make them more socially confident, it also helps them to be less anxious if you suffer a relapse and they are cared for by other people.

Local mother-and-toddler groups can offer great support as well as reassurance. When you get chatting to other mums, you may see that what you had assumed were problems related to your MS are actually stumbling blocks for *all* mothers – tiredness, stress, anxiety and so on. Gradually, as you get to know the different women, you are likely to form a support network, taking it in turns to babysit so that you each get a night out with your partners, going to infant massage classes together, and taking the children to the local park on sunny afternoons. It's far from unusual to make life-long friends at such groups.

The MS father

Being the father and having MS can be just as difficult as being the mother. In truth, whether it is the father or the mother who has the disorder, the whole family is affected. An MS father, however, can feel he is failing abysmally at being the strong, supportive head of the family. Be reassured, though, that a small child will be happy so long as you are able to spend quality time together, and so long as you are able to show love and affection.

Where your partner is concerned, she knew before she was pregnant that you had MS and that it comes with limitations. She may sometimes need a little more emotional support than before – but all it generally takes is for her to know that you are on her side. Where practical help is concerned, getting the help of family and friends can make all the difference. If you don't have help, it's possible for your wife to become resentful of your physical disabilities.

Also, you may worry about the state of your health in your child's older years – but it's really not worth it. You will always be your child's father whatever disabilities you have. As long as you continue to give time and show love and affection, all should be well in the end.

The child

It is only natural to worry about not being able to go camping with your child in summer, to play rough and tumble games on the floor, or football in the back garden. Your child may indeed miss out on certain things, but this doesn't mean his or her upbringing will be less satisfactory than the norm. Explain to your child why you can't do certain things, in language he or she will understand, and you will be surprised by how practical he or she is about it – the younger you tell them, the better it is. Children who are not told what is happening, usually in the hope of protecting them, can feel very anxious. They know something is not quite right with Mum or Dad and can worry that it is worse than it actually is. They may even believe they are a burden, a duty you could do without. Some children are convinced that it is their fault that their parent is ill and feel enormously guilty. There is no doubt at all in psychologists' minds that a child should be kept informed. Children can take on board fairly complicated concepts at a remarkably young age.

Depending on the personality and nature of the child involved, he or she may do everything possible to help or, at the other end of the spectrum, feel embarrassed or ashamed of your condition, complaining that so-and-so's mother can take her swimming and dancing and that you can do nothing. Such children are obviously frustrated that their parent cannot do what other parents do, but they are also likely to be harbouring a deep fear of what will become of their beloved Mum or Dad, which gets translated into anger. It is best for all concerned that you open up, be totally honest about your disappointments and frustrations, particularly regarding interactions with your child. Then remind your child of all the things you *can* do together. He or she should start then to see the situation differently.

Children definitely respond better when kept informed. However, it is important that they are not treated like miniature adults and have the weight of the world on their shoulders. It is also important that they do no more than light household chores. They are still children and should not be expected to do the lion's share of the work. If they are happy and know they are loved, most children will try to give as much help as is reasonable. If they kick up a fuss about performing the smallest of tasks, simply be firm. It is normal for children to be lazy and to try to wriggle out of doing work. At all costs, avoid making the child feel he or she is uncaring and insensitive for only doing what comes naturally.

7

Diet in MS

For a number of people with MS, eating the type of foods that early man ate can halt the progression of the condition. For others, these foods will have little or no influence on the advancement of the disease. There appear to be several possible triggers for MS, and dietary factors are only one of them. Having said that, each person with MS should make every effort to preserve his or her general health, and this can be achieved largely by eating wisely. Improving your diet will give you more energy, more stamina and more resistance to infections. The Paleolithic Diet, outlined below, is outstandingly healthy and should not offend even the most temperamental of digestive systems.

The Paleolithic Diet

There are groups of people who are virtually free from diseases such as cancer, arthritis, heart disease, diabetes, high blood pressure, stroke, schizophrenia and depression. These people belong to the last hunter-gatherer tribes on the planet, and eat a diet that has changed very little since the first humans evolved. This diet is known as the 'Paleolithic Diet'. It is also known as the 'Hunter-Gatherer Diet', the 'Stone-Age Diet', 'Cave-Man Diet' or the 'Best Bet Diet'.

The Paleolithic Diet comprises all the foods that were available to early man, and ignores those that weren't. It contains all the major food groups and dietary components, and because our genetic structure has evolved with a need for these early foods, this diet is compatible with our genetic make-up. When 'newer' foods are eaten, toxicity builds up and the body becomes sluggish – both for people with health conditions and those who are healthy. That's why detox diets have become so popular of late.

MS is widely accepted as being an autoimmune disorder. This means the immune system attacks the myelin sheaths that protect the nerve cells in the central nervous system. What we don't yet know is exactly what triggers the process. Researchers have theorized, however, that dietary factors are the main feature in the onset and progression of the disease, the assumption being that a failure of the digestive system activates the immune system into attacking the central nervous system. This process is termed 'leaky gut'.

Leaky gut

In a healthy person, food is thoroughly digested, broken down into miniscule units before being absorbed through the bowel wall and into the bloodstream. Our immune systems do not recognize these units as foreign because our bodies are made of the same basic building blocks as the food we eat. However, when the gut wall is significantly damaged, molecules of intact food proteins from undigested foods are able to escape into the bloodstream. Damage to the gut wall can be caused by allergenic foods, candida overgrowth, infection, parasites, stress, trauma, alcohol consumption and the use of non-steroidal anti-inflammatory drugs such as aspirin.

Because they are larger than normal, the escaped molecules (macro-molecules) are recognized as foreign by the immune system, which reacts by setting up antibodies to fight them. When vast amounts of macro-molecules are absorbed into the bloodstream, the immune system – confused by the constant onslaught – begins to attack the body's own cells by mistake. These cells can be muscles, ligaments or, in the case of MS, the myelin that protects nerve cells in the central nervous system. The immune system attacking the body's own cells is termed an 'autoimmune reaction'.

Self-proteins

The immune system can also be activated by molecular similarities between particular food proteins and proteins that exist naturally in the central nervous system – known as 'self-proteins'. When food proteins mimic self-proteins, they are able to gain access into the central nervous system through what is known as the 'blood-brain barrier', a defence system that normally stops foreign agents from reaching the central nervous system, located in the brain and spinal cord (see Chapter 1). Hypersensitivity reactions within the body – caused by foods that the digestive system is unable to tolerate – are also thought to aid the passage of food proteins into the central nervous system.

Preventing the autoimmune response

Dr Embry, a research scientist who looked closely into the effects of different foods in MS, discovered that to prevent the damaging autoimmune reaction, it is necessary to halt leaky gut and stop the consumption of foods containing proteins that mimic self-proteins existing naturally in the central nervous system. He resolved also that the blood-brain barrier and the immune system are capable of being strengthened by the use of dietary supplements. He devised the Paleolithic Diet.

Lack of sunshine

In constructing his diet, Dr Embry, like researchers before him, considered the distribution of MS and observed that the spread of the condition can clearly be seen in large countries like Australia, Canada and the USA. For instance, there is a high incidence of MS in the northern regions of countries in the northern hemisphere (Canada and the USA), where there are fewer hours of sunshine. Likewise, in Australia there is a high incidence of MS in the southern regions, where again there is less sunshine. All areas in these countries with more hours of sunshine have a lower incidence of MS. A link between MS and lack of sunshine is therefore strongly suggested.

This does not explain, however, why the number of MS cases per head of population is low in some areas with comparatively less sunshine. Studies have shown, though, that these areas have communities whose diet is based primarily on fish. As sunshine and oily fish are the two main sources of Vitamin D, it is believed that this vitamin may offer protection for those who are exposed to a lot of sunshine and eat a lot of fish. It is also believed that people who live in sunny climes and eat a lot of fish are less likely to develop MS.

Stopping self-proteins entering the central nervous system

If you would like to try Dr Embry's Paleolithic Diet, follow the instructions given in this section. The foods suspected of mimicking the molecular structure of self-proteins (see above) are listed below. In the main, they are to be avoided:

- *Dairy products:* including animal milk, butters, cheeses and yoghurts made with products that contain 'suspect' foods. Rice milk and low-fat coconut milk are good replacements for animal milk. Soya milk should be avoided as it is derived from a type of pulse (see below).
- *Gluten:* wheat, rye and barley, and all products containing these grains. Oats should also be avoided, despite evidence suggesting they are gluten-free. They are a modern grain and the risk of autoimmune reaction is less if they are excluded from the diet. Replace all the above grains with rice, corn, bran, millet, flax (linseeds), couscous and quinoa. There are also a variety of gluten-free grains and flours available in health food shops and some supermarkets.
- *Legumes:* beans, peas and pulses, especially soya. However, you can eat all other vegetables, particularly green leafy ones such as spinach and broccoli as they are high in essential omega 3 oils.
- *Refined sugar and margarine:* instead use honey, maple syrup, fructose (sugar from fruit) and stevia (a non-toxic herbal sweetener).
- *Eggs and yeast:* it is safe to eat eggs and yeast if you limit the quantities – that is, no more than three eggs a week, and no more than one small loaf of gluten-free bread. Other yeast products to cut down on include Marmite, Bovril, Vegemite, vinegar, stock cubes, soya sauce and tartare sauce.
- *Saturated fats (see below):* limit saturated fat to 15 g per day.

The Elisa test

An Elisa blood test for determining food allergies is recommended in MS as it can show whether foods have escaped through a leaky gut in the past. If leaky gut is present in the blood taken from your finger, an IgG antibody will be found. The existence of this antibody indicates that you are hypersensitive to the foods mentioned above, and food hypersensitivity contributes to the porous nature of the gut. Avoidance of the above foods for several months will give your leaky gut time to repair itself.

There are several other 'food intolerance' tests, such as muscle tests (kinesiology) and pulse tests, each of which can be criticized if one deliberately sets out to do so. The only certain way to prove the case for food sensitivities is via a food elimination programme.

A food elimination programme

Perhaps the most reliable method of establishing leaky gut is to monitor your reactions to particular foods. As this involves eliminating the suspect foods, then reintroducing them one at a time, it is time-consuming and difficult to stick to. You may wish to give it a go, however.

First, eliminate all suspect foods from your diet – dairy products, gluten, legumes, refined sugar and margarine, eggs, yeast and saturated fat – for a period of one month. (See page 78 for foods you can eat.) There may be an initial withdrawal reaction, such as fatigue, headaches, twitching and irritability, and this can last for up to 15 days. Drinking at least 4 pints (2 litres) of water each day will dramatically reduce these symptoms. This also aids detoxification and helps to flush any residual offending foods through the system. A hypersensitive stage can follow this period. If you unwittingly eat a food you are attempting to eliminate, the ensuing reaction can be severe. Dining out can be a problem, too. Ask the chef, not the waiter, if you are unsure about ingredients.

On a brighter note, a pleasing withdrawal symptom for some people can be a loss of weight. The reason for this – assuming you are not starving yourself, which would be completely wrong and unnecessary – is that many people with food sensitivities have an excess of fluid distributed throughout their bodies. When they begin to eliminate suspect foods, the excess fluid quickly drains away.

Food reintroduction strategy

When the month is up, follow the reintroduction strategy below:

Day 1: In the morning, reintroduce a small amount of dairy food – not a full-sized portion. Do the same later in the day and record your response. If you experience an adverse reaction, you know you are hypersensitive to this food and it should be withdrawn from your diet.

Day 2: If you do not experience any symptoms, repeat the exercise. Once again, record any symptoms. There must be two days without symptoms before you can safely reintroduce this food into your diet on a regular basis. However, if dairy products were indeed involved in your leaky gut problem, on its reintroduction you will experience a headache, or stomach irritations (abdominal cramps, perhaps accompanied by diarrhoea), or indigestion. An 'intolerance' response of this kind is the red flag warning that dairy produce should be withdrawn from your diet.

One week later: At this stage, you should reintroduce a small amount of gluten into your diet. If, having done so, you experience an intolerance response of the kind mentioned above, the gluten should be withdrawn. Now reintroduce the remaining foods, one at a time, and measure your body's reaction. Eliminate the offending foods from your diet for the time being. It may be possible to reintroduce them after a period of six months, when your leaky gut has had time to heal. However, some foods will always cause an adverse reaction, so it would be wise to withdraw them from your diet altogether.

You can help your leaky gut to heal by using the following supplements: acidophilus, glutathione, glutamine, grape seed extract, evening primrose oil, fish oil and digestive enzymes. As some of these supplements may interact with others, it is recommended that you ask a trained herbalist or nutritionist for advice.

Foods you can eat

- Chicken (only cooked breast, without the skin).
- Turkey (only cooked breast, without the skin).
- Liver.
- Fish.
- Wild game.
- All fruits.
- All vegetables (remember that peas and beans are legumes and should be avoided).
- Some nuts and seeds.

- Rice, corn, millet, flax (linseed), bran, quinoa and other gluten-free grains.

A low-fat diet

In his 1993 book *Fats that Heal, Fats that Kill*, Udo Erasmus wrote about the ability of fats and oils to both whip up and control inflammatory immune reactions. Research has shown that fats and oils do indeed have this capacity.

There are two distinct types of fat:

Saturated fat

This type of fat is capable of promoting an inflammatory reaction. It is derived mainly from animal sources and is generally solid at room temperature. Although margarine was, for many years, believed to be a healthier choice over butter, nutritionists have now revised their opinion, because some of the fats in the margarine hydrogenation process are changed into trans-fatty acids that the body metabolizes as if they were saturated fatty acids – the same as butter. Butter is a valuable source of oils and Vitamin A, but should be used very sparingly. Margarine, on the other hand, is an artificial product containing many additives. In MS, it is important to keep your intake of saturated fat down to less than 15 g a day. This means that all red meat and the dark meat from chicken and turkey should be avoided.

Unsaturated fat

Also called polyunsaturated or monounsaturated fat, unsaturated fat is capable of moderating an inflammatory reaction. It also has a protective effect on the organs of the body. Omega 3 and Omega 6 oils occur naturally in oily fish (mackerel, herring, salmon, sardines, fresh tuna, etc.), nuts and seeds, and is usually liquid at room temperature. It is recommended that people with MS eat oily fish at least three times a week and cold-pressed oil (olive, rapeseed, safflower and sunflower oil) daily, both in dressings and in cooking. Olive oil is best suited to cooking, however, as it suffers less damage from heat than other oils. In a 1996 study, after a low incidence of inflammatory bowel disease was reported in Eskimos, fish oil was found to be very beneficial in controlling Crohn's disease – another autoimmune dysfunction (Belluzzi *et al.*, 1996). A maximum consumption of 60 g daily of unsaturated fat is recommended in MS.

Strengthening the blood-brain barrier

When the immune system is activated by undigested food molecules or food proteins that mimic self-proteins (ones that occur naturally in the body), the blood–brain barrier is breached and damaged. Experiments have shown that the chemicals occurring naturally in blueberries (bilberries), cherries, blackberries, grapes and the bark and needles of a particular pine tree are able to strengthen the blood-brain barrier. If you are unable to eat a significant amount of the above, supplements should be taken every day. Other supplements that can have a beneficial effect on the blood-brain barrier – although not so powerful as the above – are antioxidants, Vitamin A, Vitamin C (with bioflavonoids) and Vitamin E. Along with Vitamin B complex and Vitamin D, these supplements should, ideally, be taken daily in MS.

Nutritional supplements

In MS, the immune system can be strengthened – and suppressed where necessary – by the following supplements. The dosages given are too low to cause toxicity problems. You should only exceed these dosages on your doctor's advice.

Of course, to purchase all of the following every month would be very expensive. Buy what you can afford and remember that every little helps.

The recommended daily supplements are as follows:

- Vitamin D. Ask your doctor for a blood test (the 25(OH)D test which is generally free in the UK) to determine your requirement of this particular vitamin. There is no single supplement dosage that will help you to reach the optimum level. Some people can take 4000 iu all year round, but others need to take only 1000 iu. The test should then be carried out every six months, in April and October, to ensure that you stay within the optimum levels.
- Grape seed extract – 300 mg. (Use pycnogenol or bilberry if you have an intolerance to grapes.)

- Cod liver oil – 2 g. (This includes 5,000 iu of Vitamin A and 400 iu of Vitamin D.)
- Salmon oil – 4 g.
- High-strength Vitamin B complex – 2 tablets or capsules.
- Vitamin B12 – 100 mcg.
- Vitamin C – 3 g.
- Vitamin E – 800 iu.
- Calcium – 1500 mg. (It's recommended that you avoid dairy products completely, so you will need this alternative form of calcium.)
- Magnesium – 750 mg. (The optimum ratio for calcium versus magnesium is 2 to 1.)
- Zinc – 25 mg.
- Copper – 2 mg.
- Selenium – 50 mcg.
- Evening primrose oil or borage oil – 5 g.
- Flaxseed oil – 10 g. (Be careful to note whether you have an intolerance to flax before taking this.)
- Acidophilus – 4 capsules.
- Digestive enzymes – 6 capsules.
- Lecithin – 2400 mg.

The Paleolithic Diet in brief

It is suggested that people with MS do the following:

- Drink 4 pints (2 litres) of water a day.
- Avoid drinks containing caffeine, such as coffee, tea, hot chocolate and cola drinks. Caffeine is dehydrating, and cutting it out may help people with urge incontinence.
- Ensure your diet is high in fibre, particularly from whole grains. The best fibre foods are bran, oats and flax (linseed).
- Eat plenty of fruit, particularly prunes, as they can ease constipation.
- Eat plenty of vegetables.
- Eat fish and skinless breast of chicken and turkey.
- Avoid red meat.
- Try to eat a low-fat diet. Studies have shown no real benefit on the disease process for eating a low-fat diet – however, it will help to improve your general health.

- Avoid saturated fats. These include margarine, lard, cream and other fats that are solid at room temperature. Use butter sparingly.
- Eat plenty of unsaturated fats. These include olives and olive oil, canola oil, oils with high levels of oleic acid, rapeseed oil, safflower oil, cornflower oil, flaxseed oil, avocados, nuts and seeds.
- Avoid dairy products, gluten and legumes, unless the Elisa blood test shows they are not causing a problem.
- If the Elisa test is not available to you, use the food elimination programme to test whether you are hypersensitive to particular foods. If you find that you are, cut them out of your diet for a period of six months, after which you may be able to slowly reintroduce them. Some foods, though, may always be a problem.
- Avoid soya products.
- Eat nuts and seeds as snacks.
- Eat oily fish. These include mackerel, herring, sardines and fresh tuna.
- Take as many of the recommended supplements (listed above) as your budget allows.

So what can I eat for breakfast?

If you wish to eliminate dairy produce, gluten and legumes from your diet, you should be able to replace them with the following:

- Kiwi, grapefruit, bananas and other fruits in season. Put different fruits in a blender with a little orange juice to make a nutritious drink.
- Pancakes made with gluten-free flour, served with honey or maple syrup.
- Grilled kippers with grilled tomatoes and mushrooms.
- Fresh fruit salad.
- Gluten-free toasted bread with sardines.
- A large wedge of cantaloupe melon.
- Toasted rice bread, spread with honey or mashed banana.
- Rice cakes.
- Try making your own muesli with a mixture of puffed rice, sunflower seeds, linseeds, sesame seeds, millet, dried dates, raisins, hazelnuts and toasted pumpkin seeds. Pour on hot or cold rice milk before eating.

So what can I eat for lunch?

Here are a few suggestions for lunch:

- Jacket potato with cottage cheese and pineapple or onion, with an avocado salad, followed by a banana.
- Vegetable soup, followed by rice cakes.
- Chicken or turkey breast sandwich, made with gluten-free bread, followed by an orange.
- Peanut butter sandwiches, assuming you are not allergic to peanuts, followed by baked apples with honey.
- Tuna salad, followed by a slice of melon.
- Salad with roll-mops (marinated fillets of herring wrapped around pickled onions or other vegetables), followed by banana muffins (made with gluten-free flour).

So what can I eat for dinner?

Here are a few suggestions:

- Baked wild salmon with potatoes, broccoli and carrots.
- Mixed vegetable casserole with millet.
- Grilled turkey breast with potatoes, cauliflower and sage and onion stuffing.
- Broiled fish (any kind) with steamed vegetables.
- Tuna, spinach and pasta bake, using gluten-free pasta.
- Chicken curry with brown rice (using only chicken breast).
- Grilled mackerel with potatoes, cabbage and carrots.
- Falafel (similar to a veggie burger and available from health food shops) with delicious home-made chips (brush with olive oil and oven-bake), onion rings and grilled tomatoes.

Eating out

Don't be afraid to ask for what you want, and the way you want it cooked. If you are hypersensitive to dairy foods and gluten, tell the waiter. You might be best sticking to a salad or grilled fish/chicken or turkey breast meat with a jacket potato. For a special meal where you want to be more adventurous, ring ahead and explain to the chef that you can't eat certain foods. Given sufficient time, the chef will no doubt be pleased to prepare you a dish you can eat with both safety and relish!

8

Other possible causes

Because MS is one of the most complex conditions to affect the human body, the full picture of its cause is not yet clear. To date, the leading theory is that MS is triggered by a viral infection in people who carry the MS gene. An infection is suspected because the central nervous system lesions and increased levels of a chemical called IgG are characteristic of a particular infectious disorder, as shown by Bansil *et al.* in a 1994 study. Several other studies – of twins, animals and human subjects – have indicated that MS is generally virally induced.

One study of identical and fraternal twins, also conducted by Bansil *et al.*, suggested that the susceptibility to MS was much greater in identical twins – 31 per cent in identical twins compared with 5 per cent in fraternal twins. This proves a strong genetic link. Studies of twins have also shown that external factors can play a major role in the development of MS.

Infectious agents

Studies suggest that infectious agents, most probably viruses, are likely to play a large part in the onset of MS. The reasons for this belief are as follows:

- Four separate clusters of MS outbreaks arose between 1943 and 1989 in the Faroe Islands, which are located between Iceland and Scandinavia. The islands were occupied by British troops during the First World War, after which the incidence of MS increased yearly for 20 years. Researchers concluded that the troops might have brought with them a disease-causing agent.
- Some viruses are strikingly similar to the proteins in myelin and may therefore confuse the immune system, causing T-cells to attack the body's own protein rather than the viral agent. More than one agent may be involved. While some may trigger the disease, others may keep the process going.

One suspect agent is possibly an infection acquired before the age of 15. It may lie dormant in the brain until set into action in people who carry the MS gene and who have defective immune control mechanisms. When activated by one of the triggers mentioned earlier – dietary factors, stress, inhalants, heavy metals, trauma, and so on – the immune system will start to run riot and MS develops. It is theorized that the virus may be as simple and common as the following:

- The herpes virus. HHV-6, a form of herpes virus that causes roseola, a benign disease in children, is also known to cause encephalitis (inflammation of the brain) in patients with impaired immune systems. A number of studies have reported higher than normal rates of HHV-6 infection in MS patients, and some experts believe that may be an important factor in MS. Other experts argue, however, that nearly everyone harbours this virus and that there is no evidence of a causal relationship. Other herpes viruses can also infect brain cells. They include herpes simplex 1 and 2 (the causes of oral and genital herpes), varicella-zoster virus (the cause of chicken pox and shingles), and cytomegalovirus.
- *Chlamydia pneumoniae*. This is a bacterium that has been associated with persistent inflammation in small blood vessels. A few studies have reported significantly higher rates of previous Chlamydia infection in MS patients than in people without MS. An important group of studies in the year 2000, though, reported no connection at all between Chlamydia and MS. Some researchers suggest that different laboratory standards in identifying the organism have produced varying results. Many experts now believe there is no strong evidence linking the microbe to MS.

Other viruses that have been investigated include the Epstein-Barr virus (the cause of mononucleosis), the measles virus, adenovirus, polyomavirus, and the retroviruses (HIV, HTLV-I, and HTLV-II). Indeed, in one 1992 study of five people with neurological problems associated with the Epstein-Barr virus, four went on to develop acute MS within 4–12 years of contracting the infection (Bray *et al.*, 1992).

A virus works by infecting the cells and, after multiplying, causes the cells to die. The immune system then attacks and destroys the virus. Certain common viruses (some of which are mentioned above) are capable of entering the brain, and once there they cause inflammation and demyelination. However, the immune system quietens down the inflammation, after which damage to the myelin or myelin-producing cells is slowly reversed. When a component of the myelin resembles the virus, or if the virus itself remains dormant in the brain, the immune system may mistakenly attack the brain. There have been unverified reports of researchers finding evidence of virus particles in some people with MS. Scientific evidence for a definite link with infections and MS is now being sought.

Where relapses of MS are concerned, there is strong evidence that certain viral infections may provoke them.

Dietary factors

Experts believe that food intolerances and other dietary factors may be the trigger for MS in a large number of cases. Avoiding suspect foods and eating a more basic diet, boosted by nutritional supplements, can ease symptoms and either slow or halt the disease progression. Dietary factors are discussed in detail in Chapter 7.

Inhalants

Inhalants such as cigarette smoke, car exhaust fumes, household chemicals, lawn and garden sprays and so on are thought to be a possible cause of immune system reactions which activate T-cells and lead to the demyelination of nerve cells. The person doesn't need to have an obvious adverse reaction to be sensitive to inhalants. There is an allergy test called Elisa (see Chapter 7) that measures a person's response to a variety of inhalants and can therefore specify whether they play a major role in their MS. If the test is positive, it is essential to cut down your exposure to these substances, but this may prove difficult. It may be necessary for you to move to a different area, or even to a different country where the air is cleaner.

Heavy metals

Heavy metals can be toxic to the central nervous system and may contribute to the onset of MS. Unfortunately, our bodies are absorbing small quantities of heavy metals every day. Hair mineral analysis, carried out through a qualified nutritionist, can show the levels of minerals in the body. The worst culprits are aluminium, mercury and lead:

- *Aluminium:* Sources of aluminium poisoning may be aluminium saucepans, foil and foil containers and underarm deodorants. This metal can also be found in coffee, bleached white flour and some antacid medications. Experts now believe that magnesium and calcium deficiencies increase the toxic effects of ingested aluminium.
- *Mercury:* People with amalgam tooth fillings are ingesting minute amounts of mercury vapour every day, and mercury is the second most toxic heavy metal in the world. There is no evidence of a higher incidence of MS in people with mercury fillings, and there are plenty of people without such fillings who have MS. However, there is sufficient theoretical data available to indicate that mercury fillings are capable of causing the progression of MS. Synthetic white fillings are a safe alternative.
- *Lead:* Ingested lead can cause damage to the central nervous system and ultimately lead to psychological disturbances. Some old houses still have lead piping, others have copper piping fused together with lead-based solder. The use of a jug water-filter is highly recommended in cases like this – although, obviously, replacing the old piping with modern copper or synthetic piping is far safer.

Vaccinations

Adverse reactions involving the central nervous system have been reported from a variety of different vaccinations. It would appear that, in some cases, vaccinations can cause inflammation of the central nervous system and result in the demyelination of the nerves. In fact, there are numerous reports suggesting that both onset and worsening of MS may occur following a vaccination. Dr Charles Poser has postulated that the vaccination is often the final straw to an already stressed immune system. Indeed, he is able to give details of cases where vaccinations lead to the onset of MS.

Concerns about a link between the hepatitis B vaccine and MS led

France to stop a major vaccination programme in 1998. Subsequent research published in 2001, however, found no evidence of any causal link, and studies have indicated that the influenza vaccination is safe in MS. Despite that, experts advise that if you are considering the flu jab, you should only have it if absolutely necessary.

Other possible triggers

There are several other possible triggers for MS. They include the following:

- *Trauma:* Some experts believe that injury (trauma) to the head, neck, or upper back may trigger MS by disrupting the blood–brain barrier and allowing entry to the attacking immune system into the central nervous system. There is little supporting evidence for this theory, however.
- *Stress:* Stress is not believed to be a cause of MS, but the connection between stress and an exacerbation of symptoms is very well known. Stress is believed to trigger the disease in susceptible people.
- *Cows' milk for babies rather than breast milk:* As mentioned in Chapter 6, there is some evidence that infants fed only on cows' milk may have a higher than average risk of developing MS in adulthood. Breast milk, on the other hand, contains factors that may help to regulate the immune response. However, not all cows' milk is the same, and it appears that some milk proteins carry higher risks than others.
- *Other foreign matter:* The statements of 26 women with failed silicone breast implants give a vivid insight into what can happen when toxins reach the central nervous system. Each woman had central nervous system lesions, as shown on MRI scans – caused by demyelination of the nerves. There was also evidence of inflammatory autoimmune disease, triggered by the foreign material in their bodies.

9

Complementary therapies

Research has shown that almost 60 per cent of people with MS try complementary therapies. You may know these as 'alternative therapies' – but this term can be misleading. The word 'alternative' suggests that the therapy can be used to replace conventional medicine. Unfortunately, in treating MS this is not the case.

There is little research on the usefulness of complementary therapies in MS, and there are known to be possible adverse reactions to some types. Some studies show benefits from using a certain therapy, but the compound used in the studies may not be what is marketed to the public – their quality and strength is not controlled by a regulating body. Before deciding to try a particular therapy, it is recommended that you find out as much as you can about it. You could also ask your doctor's advice.

Some people with MS who use complementary therapies report great benefits. However, the benefits may, to some extent, come from knowing they are doing something positive to help themselves. Different therapies appear to suit different people.

Acupuncture

An ancient form of oriental healing, acupuncture involves puncturing the skin with fine needles at specific points in the body. These points are located along energy channels (meridians) which are believed to correspond with certain internal organs. This energy is known as chi. Needles are inserted to increase, decrease or unblock the flow of chi energy so that the balance of yin and yang is restored. It is thought that an imbalance in these forces is the cause of illness and disease.

Acupuncture has been used to alleviate stress, digestive disorders, insomnia, asthma and allergies. Studies have shown that treatment prompts the brain to release both endorphins and encephalins (natural painkillers), strengthen the immune system and calm the nervous system.

A qualified acupuncturist will use a set method to determine acupuncture points – it is thought there are as many as 2,000 on the body. At a consultation, questions may be asked about lifestyle, sleeping patterns, fears, phobias, and reactions to stress. The pulses will be felt, then the acupuncture itself carried out, with fine needles being placed in the relevant sites. The first consultation will normally last an hour, and patients should feel improvements after four to six sessions.

Although acupuncture is losing its unorthodox reputation, it is still viewed with scepticism by a large part of the medical profession. However, some doctors have great respect for the benefits of acupuncture and even perform the therapy themselves.

Some studies have shown that acupuncture triggers the release of certain proteins in the central nervous system, which can reduce some MS symptoms. Acupuncturists say the main aim of treatment is to maintain the person in the progressive-remitting stage for as long as possible. If the disease does progress, acupuncture aims to reduce the symptoms and keep the person from entering the next stage.

Acupuncture is a safe therapy. The only slight risk is that of infection from the needles.

Bioelectromagnetics

Bioelectromagnetics is the study of how living organisms – all of which produce electrical currents – interact with magnetic fields. The electrical currents within our bodies are capable of creating magnetic fields that extend outside our bodies, and these fields can be influenced by external magnetic forces. In fact, specific external magnetism can actually produce physical and behavioural changes. Just as drugs induce a response on their target tissues, so low magnetic fields can produce a chosen biological response – but without the chemical side-effects associated with drugs.

External magnetism can not only correct abnormalities in the energy fields of patients with disease, effectively working as a healer, it is also claimed to be capable of stabilizing a chronic condition – although it certainly doesn't do so in every case. A few small, uncontrolled studies have reported improvements in pain, fatigue, tremors and other symptoms in people severely affected with MS. As a pain reliever, external magnetism is becoming ever more widely used, and much experimentation is currently under way. Electro-magnetic machinery is even becoming a regular part of NHS treatment. The machinery creates a pulsed magnetic field which is used to aid the recovery of bone fractures, tendon and ligament tears, muscle injuries, etc. A small, light, comparatively inexpensive version of the above can be purchased for easy-to-wear home use, to help relieve the pain, tremors and fatigue of MS. External magnetism should not be used by anyone fitted with a heart pacemaker.

External magnetism in the form of a specially designed wrist appliance – worn like a wrist watch – is also believed to be effective in treating aches and pains in any region of the body. As with other types of external magnetism, this appliance is said to improve the ability of the blood to carry oxygen and nutrients around the body. It is also believed to speed the removal of toxins and other waste products. Various appliances are available for use on different parts of the body. (See the Useful addresses section at the back of this book for outlet details.)

Homeopathy

The general consensus of homeopaths is that people with MS usually respond well to homeopathic treatment, but you should consult a qualified practitioner. It is a common misconception that you can just pop along to your local chemist or health shop, look up your particular complaint on the homeopathic remedy chart, and begin taking that particular remedy. If only it were that simple! Homeopathic training takes several years, and a lot of knowledge and experience is required before practitioners can decide the correct remedies for complaints other than the very superficial. And, what works for one person is not liable to work for another.

In 1925, the homeopath to the British royal family, W. W. Rorke, reported that of seven people treated for an MS symptom, three had complete recovery, three were much improved, and the remaining person had little or no change. Dr Andre Saine reported recently that of the 22 MS cases under his care, 50 per cent had results ranging from excellent to very good, 35 per cent had results that were rated as good to fair, and 15 per cent had outcomes classed as poor to no results (six subjects were excluded as it was impossible for Saine to follow them up). The cases were a mix of mild, moderate and severe MS. These results are consistent with those reported by other homeopaths. However, they agree that a symptom that has been in existence for more than two years is difficult to reverse and that earlier, milder cases of MS respond more favourably to homeopathic treatment.

According to homeopaths, better results are seen in the northern hemisphere when treatment is administered between April and October. The reverse is the case in the southern hemisphere. It would appear that dry weather conditions are beneficial to homeopathy, while wet weather and rapid change from warm to cold and vice versa in winter can hinder treatment.

Reflexology

A small-scale study into the effects of reflexology on volunteers with MS was conducted in 1997 (Joyce *et al.*, 1997). After six weeks of treatment, improvements were reported, but during the second six-week period, some improvements were lost by several of the participants. Surprisingly, after a total of 18 weeks of treatment, improvements in 45 per cent of symptoms were reported. This suggests that reflexology does offer therapeutic effect, but primarily if treatments continue for at least 18 weeks.

In a larger MS study over a three-month period in 2003, significant improvements were reported in the scores for bladder problems, spasticity, numbness and tingling (Siev-Ner *et al.*, 2003). The reflexology group showed borderline improvement in muscle strength scores, and the improvement in numbness and tingling remained significant at a three-month follow-up. The control group – where a sham foot-massaging treatment had been given – showed no such improvements.

Reflexology is certainly relaxing. Indeed, many patients fall asleep during the therapy. Because my own feet are so ticklish, I felt I had cause to worry before my first reflexology session. (I could imagine myself involuntarily kicking the therapist!) Fortunately, I quickly found that the sensations were pleasurable and I was able to relax – and I was surprised to note how accurate the therapist was in detecting my own 'indispositions'.

Herbal remedies

Traditional Chinese herbal remedies have been used, to great effect, since antiquity – and are still the most widely used medicines in the world. In fact, 30 per cent of modern conventional medicines are made from plant-derived substances.

Although they are natural and there is a lower incidence of serious reactions than there is with Western conventional medications, herbal medicines should still be used with caution. Most are gentle and unlikely to cause serious side-effects, but because, like conventional medication, they contain physiologically active agents, side-effects can occur. The most common reactions are throat irritations, gastrointestinal upsets and headaches. You should always inform your doctor of what you are taking. Indeed, many doctors believe herbal medicine should not be taken without the advice of a trained herbalist. Your chosen herbalist will check your pulse rate and the colour of your tongue for clues as to which bodily organs are energy-depleted. They will then write a prescription for very precise dosages according to your needs. Tablets made from compressed herbal extracts are often supplied, but sometimes patients are given a bag of carefully weighed and ground dried roots, flowers, bark and so on, together with instructions.

The herbs described below are considered useful for treating MS. Please note, however, that there have never been any proper randomized scientific studies to assess their validity. Moreover, because there is often no dosage information for remedies purchased from a health shop or supermarket, it is difficult to know how much is *too much*. As well as causing side-effects, herbal remedies can interfere with prescription medication. Therefore, it is strongly recommended that you follow the advice of a trained herbalist. There are a lot of them around nowadays.

If you are taking large doses of prescription medication for severe symptoms, you may prefer to use herbal remedies for the more routine ailments you encounter.

Bilberry

This herb is claimed to enhance eye health, improve night vision and prevent macular degeneration – the macula is the region of the eye responsible for the greatest visual clarity. If you have eye problems, you may wish to try bilberry in regulated doses.

Cranberry

Because urinary tract infections can trigger relapses in MS, you may wish to drink cranberry juice, which helps to prevent such infections. Cranberry juice is thought to be safe in moderate quantities. If you take blood-thinners such as warfarin and heparin, however, avoid cranberry juice. Cartons of cranberry juice are now available in most supermarkets.

Echinacea

One of the most researched herbs, echinacea, has broad antibiotic properties, much like penicillin. It acts as an immune system stimulant, aids the destruction of germs, and is capable of strengthening cell defences. As an antiviral agent, echinacea may be used by people with MS at the first signs of a cold or flu to lessen the chances of a relapse occurring. Some people with MS have reported a reduction in all their symptoms as a result of regularly using this herb. Adverse reactions are possible, so use carefully at first to monitor the effects.

Alcohol-free echinacea tinctures are now available from most health food shops. Alternatively, dry echinacea root – also available in health food shops – can be infused to make tea.

Garlic

This herb is useful for fighting viral, bacterial and parasitic infections, so can be of great benefit in MS. Garlic pearls are available from most health food shops. However, you may prefer to use natural garlic in your cooking.

Ginkgo biloba

This herbal antioxidant is capable of boosting blood circulation. As a result, cognitive function (concentration, memory, etc.) is improved, as is energy production. In two trials undertaken in the 1990s, volunteers were given ginkgo biloba daily. One trial (Kleijjnen *et al.*, 1992) showed that the volunteers' short-term memories had improved significantly, and in the other study (Warot *et al.*, 1991) the volunteers displayed even sharper reactions and recall, as well as improved brain function – all of which were judged to be a result of the volunteers' improved circulation. Ginkgo biloba is, therefore, considered very useful in the treatment of MS.

In another study, intravenous injections of a constituent of ginkgo biloba, known as ginkgolide B, were given to people with MS for five days. Some 80 per cent reported improvements as a result. This treatment is still experimental, however.

Ginkgo biloba can be purchased in capsule form from health food shops, some pharmacies and the larger supermarkets, and the label dosage instructions should be followed. Don't take ginkgo biloba if you are on prescribed medication – that is, if you are prescribed warfarin, heparin and aspirin – as they can react adversely to this supplement.

Rhodiola rosea

This powerful Russian nutrient also belongs to the family of adaptogenic herbs. For people who feel stressed, this herb can encourage the body to adapt. Research has shown that rhodiola rosea can boost sexual function, help to raise energy levels, increase resistance to disease and aid the detoxification of hormones before they are eliminated from the body. It is also believed to have revitalizing properties and can help to stabilize mood swings.

Most health food shops now stock this stress-busting adaptogen, as do specialist supplement manufacturers. (See the Useful addresses section at the back of this book for further details.) Follow the label dosage instructions very carefully.

Ashwagandha

Also an adaptogenic herb, ashwagandha – sometimes called Indian ginseng – is an important tonic, containing a broad range of important healing powers rare in the plant kingdom. Not only is it good for restoring energy in people who often feel tired, it has also been shown in research to help to ease insomnia and stress.

In one study of 101 subjects, the indications of ageing – such as greying hair and low calcium levels – were found to be significantly improved in those taking ashwagandha (Kupparanjan *et al.*, 1980). Some 70 per cent of this study group also reported increased libido and improved sexual function.

95

Ashwagandha can be found in most health food shops and is available from specialist supplement manufacturers. Again, follow the label dosage instructions very carefully.

Siberian ginseng

The many benefits of Siberian ginseng – a very safe adaptogenic herb – are said to include increased physical endurance under stress and better sexual function. It is also used to treat fatigue, lethargy, depression and chronic infections. This stimulant herb is available from most health food shops and specialist supplement manufacturers. Follow the label dosage instructions with care.

St John's Wort

St John's Wort is probably the most successful natural antidepressant. Studies have shown that it works by increasing the action of the chemical serotonin and by inhibiting the depression-promoting enzymes. Similar effects are created by the drugs in the Prozac and Nardil families of chemical antidepressants – both of which carry a high risk of side-effects. St John's Wort, however, has the happy advantage of being virtually free of side-effects. (In some cases it can produce a stomach upset, but this should stop within a few days.)

One study has indicated that St John's Wort encourages sleep, and another that it benefits the immune system. In Germany, this herb outsells Prozac by three to one, and is said to be just as effective for treating mild depression. Because of its anti-inflammatory and antiviral properties, it can also be useful for treating MS. It helps fight viral infections, too. (Note: Because your skin may be more sensitive to the sun's rays when you are taking this herb, don't forget to use a good sun-block.)

Green tea

Because a major constituent of green tea has been found to powerfully inhibit auto-reactive immune cells, green tea is often of benefit to people with MS. Green tea is derived from dried leaves from the *Camellia sinesis* plant, which came over to the West from China 5,000 years ago. Green tea is popular for its taste, as well as its health benefits. It can be drunk with or without sugar and milk, and is available in health food shops and most supermarkets.

Bee venom

You may have heard that bee venom has been used to great effect in MS. Bee venom is certainly believed to contain anti-inflammatory properties that calm the immune system. However, stings can only be received by people who keep bees privately – such people take up to three stings a week.

It is important to note that this therapy has not been clinically tested and has no recognized medical approval. In fact, serious, even fatal, reactions can occur as a result of being stung by bees.

Cannabis (marijuana)

Also known as weed, skunk, ganja, pot, grass, green, herb and blow, cannabis has been the subject of much controversy regarding its use in MS. It is estimated that 1–4 per cent of the MS population in the UK are using cannabis in one form or another to relieve their symptoms, and there is a great deal of anecdotal evidence regarding its success.

Four small trials failed to prove its effects, so in November 2003 the largest study ever undertaken into cannabis and the treatment of symptoms in MS was conducted (Zajicek et al., 2003), using 657 MS patients with stable MS and problems with spasticity. One group took cannabis extract, the second group took THC – a major component of cannabis – and the third group took a placebo (sugar pill). Of course, no one knew what exactly they were taking. THC proved to have no significant impact on muscle spasticity, as measured by the Ashworth scale (an independent assessment of spasticity). Evidence of improved mobility was seen, however, and most of the subjects reported a reduction in the symptoms of their spasticity, including the pain. They also reported better sleep quality and fewer spasms. There was no evidence that the cannabis treatments had any effect on neurological symptoms, coping with daily living, sense of well-being and general mood. Mobility was not seen to be improved using the Rivermead Mobility Index (an independent assessment of walking ability), but walking time over a 10-metre distance improved by 12 per cent. Moreover, fewer relapses occurred in the groups taking whole cannabis extract and THC than in the control group. This particular study raised the question of whether the Ashworth scale is sufficiently sensitive to detect small but significant changes. Researchers concluded that cannabinoids, the active chemicals in cannabis, may be useful in treating some MS symptoms, but that further research is required.

In the UK, it's still illegal to use cannabis, so the drug cannot be prescribed. The Alliance for Cannabis Therapeutics is campaigning for changes in the law. When illegally grown in the UK, cannabis is almost always chemically accelerated at a super-fast rate, under 12-hour ultraviolet lights in a secret room. As a result, it is far stronger than that grown legally, under natural conditions, in the fields of the Netherlands, for example. Until cannabis is legalized in the UK – if ever – its use cannot be condoned.

Relaxation and meditation

You may wonder how relaxation techniques and meditation can help a person with MS. Well, stress is a common trigger of MS relapses. Therefore, avoiding it can have great benefits for your well-being and overall health.

Deep breathing

When we are stressed or upset, we tend to use the rib muscles to expand the chest. We breathe more quickly, sucking in shallowly. This is good in a crisis as it allows us to obtain the optimum amount of oxygen in the shortest possible time, providing our bodies with the extra power needed to handle the emergency. Some people do tend to get stuck in chest-breathing mode, however. Long-term shallow breathing is not only detrimental to physical and emotional health, it can also lead to hyperventilation, panic attacks, chest pains, dizziness and gastrointestinal problems.

To test your breathing, ask yourself:

- How fast are you breathing as you are reading this?
- Are you pausing between breaths?
- Are you breathing with your chest or with your diaphragm?

A breathing exercise

The following deep breathing exercise should, ideally, be performed daily:

1 Lie down in a warm room where you know you will be alone for at least half an hour.

2 Close your eyes and try to relax.
3 Gradually slow down your breathing – inhaling and exhaling as evenly as possible.
4 Place one hand on your chest and the other on your abdomen, just below your rib-cage.
5 As you inhale, allow your abdomen to swell up and out. (Your chest should barely move.)
6 As you exhale, let your abdomen flatten.

Give yourself a few minutes to get into a smooth, easy rhythm. As worries and distractions arise, don't hang on to them. Wait calmly for them to float out of your mind – then focus once more on your breathing.

When you feel ready to end the exercise, open your eyes. Allow yourself time to become alert before rolling on to one side and getting up. With practice, you will begin breathing with your diaphragm quite naturally – and in times of stress, you should be able to correct your breathing without too much effort.

A relaxation exercise

Relaxation is one of the forgotten skills in today's hectic world, but it can help to counter the effects of stress. It is advisable, therefore, that you learn at least one relaxation technique. The following exercise is perhaps the easiest:

1 Make yourself comfortable in a place where you will not be disturbed. (Listening to restful music may help you to relax.)
2 Begin to slow down your breathing, inhaling through your nose to a count of two.
3 Ensuring that the abdomen pushes outwards (as explained above), exhale to a count of four, five or six.
4 After a couple of minutes, concentrate on each part of your body in turn, starting with your right arm. Consciously relax each set of muscles, allowing the tension to flow right out. Let your arm feel heavier and heavier as every last remnant of tension seeps away. Follow this procedure with the muscles of your left arm, then the muscles of your face, your neck, your stomach, your hips, and finally your legs.

Visualization

At this point, visualization can be introduced into the exercise. As you continue to breathe slowly and evenly, imagine yourself surrounded, perhaps, by lush, peaceful countryside, beside a gently trickling stream – or maybe on a deserted tropical beach, beneath swaying palm fronds, listening to the sounds of the ocean, thousands of miles from your worries and cares. Let the warm sun, the gentle breeze, the peacefulness of it all, wash over you.

The tranquillity you feel at this stage can be enhanced by repeating the exercise frequently – once or twice a day is best. With time, you should be able to switch into a calm state of mind whenever you feel stressed.

Meditation

Arguably the oldest natural therapy, meditation is the simplest and most effective form of self-help. Dr Herbert Benson of Harvard Medical School has shown that meditation tends to normalize blood pressure, the pulse rate and level of stress hormones in the blood. He has proven, too, that it produces changes in brain wave patterns, showing less excitability, and that it strengthens the immune system and endocrine system (hormones).

The unusual thing about meditation is that it involves 'letting go', allowing the mind to roam freely. Most of us are used to trying to control our thoughts – in our work, for example – so letting go is not so easy as it sounds.

It may help to know that people who regularly meditate say they have more energy, require less sleep, are less anxious, and feel far more 'alive' than before they did so. Ideally, the technique should be taught by a teacher – but, as meditation is essentially performed alone, it can be learned on one's own with equal success.

Close your eyes, relax, and practise the deep breathing exercise as described.

1 Concentrate on your breathing. Try to free your mind of conscious control.
2 Letting your thoughts roam unchecked, try to allow the deeper, more serene part of you to take over.
3 If you wish to go further into meditation, concentrate now on

mentally repeating a 'mantra' – a certain word or phrase. It should be something positive, such as 'relax', 'I feel calm', 'I am feeling much better', or even 'I am special'.

4 When you are ready to finish, open your eyes and allow time to adjust to the outside world before standing up.

The aim of mentally repeating a mantra is to plant positive thoughts into your subconscious mind. It is a form of self-hypnosis, and you alone control the messages placed there.

10

Emotional help

Until you have a diagnosis, the most natural thing in the world is to be sick with fear and dread and to feel you're balanced on the edge of a precipice – a nudge this way and you're safe, a nudge that way and you're over. Life is on hold until you know the truth. Yet a large part of you doesn't want to know, doesn't want to have to face the possibility of your life being ripped apart by disease.

During this twilight period, some people try very hard to keep busy, while others are so stricken with anxiety they can barely function. If you are waiting for final test results, that date on the calendar might seem like the end of life as you know it. It is certainly a day you hope will never arrive, yet it seems to be rushing forward with alarming speed.

After the diagnosis

Few people with MS will forget exactly where they were, when, and with whom on the day they received their diagnosis. Being told you have MS is news that would put anyone into a state of shock and imprint that day on your mind for all eternity, even though you may have tried to be prepared for the worst.

Your anger may be almost paralysing at times – anger at your doctors, at the illness, at its ability to frighten you like this, and at your inability to understand what is happening to your body. This is normal, however, as is the feeling of unreality, of being alone, and of being tainted in some way. On top of that, your family seems to be needing reassurance from you as much as you need it from them – and, worse still, you feel they are looking at you differently. Then there are others who simply cannot understand your fears, who find it impossible to put themselves in another person's shoes.

Some newly diagnosed people react by distancing themselves emotionally from others, confiding only in the people very close to them, maybe even carrying on as normal on the surface. Others react by gathering close all the people they know and love, extracting what comfort they can from as many outstretched arms as possible. It all depends on your particular personality.

How you receive the diagnosis

Ideally, a person is given the diagnosis from a trusted doctor or neurologist, with just the right mix of compassion and encouragement. It is when you are told in an offhand manner by someone brusque and unsympathetic that the shock and fear can be both profound and devastating. Some people find out by accident on glimpsing their medical notes, or they peek at their notes themselves, or are informed in error by a medical professional who assumed they already knew, or are told by relatives who don't really understand the condition. Obviously, when discovered by such means, the news can be traumatic. If you have learnt of your MS in such a way, it is advised that you ask for an immediate referral to a recommended neurologist so you can speak about all your concerns.

Returning to your neurologist

As a rule, when most people look back on the appointment that brought their diagnosis, they remember only the jumble of emotions they experienced at the time. The doctor or neurologist might have explained what could happen in the future; he or she might have carefully relayed all your treatment options, yet the only words you heard were, 'You have multiple sclerosis.' If this happened to you and you're still not entirely clear about something, don't hesitate to make a second appointment. Neurologists in particular will understand that you didn't take everything in and will be only too happy to repeat all the information and advice they gave.

On this visit, be prepared. Write down all your questions and concerns – they may include things like, 'What do I do if I get a new symptom?' 'What do I do if I have a relapse?' and 'What do I do if the first medication doesn't suit me?' Take your pen and notepad and make notes throughout the appointment. It wouldn't be out of order for you to actually 'interview' the neurologist – after all, besides being paid to help you, neurologists experience great feelings of satisfaction when they are able to answer all your questions.

A new start

It is only when you have all the information that you can start slowly to put the pieces together, to see the complete picture of what's been happening to your body of late. The numbness you felt in your foot one day now makes sense, as does that tingling you have been experiencing in your jaw and the weird vision in your right eye on occasion. In reality, these symptoms were already the start of your new life – a life with MS – only you didn't yet know it. Now is the time to put your old life aside and try facing up to your new life. If you're the type of person who enjoys a challenge, then adjusting might not be too difficult. However, if you are quite fearful of change, you may find it more difficult to adapt. You may surprise yourself, though. Learning to live with MS is going to be the challenge of your life – and you may find that in general you cope very well.

In the early days after diagnosis, it may seem that your world has been turned upside down. And it has. The beginnings of reactive depression may then overlay all the other negative emotions flying around in your head. Add to that the onset of symptoms – whether existing or new – and it can seem like you are not the same person any more, that you have a different identity altogether.

It's not 'the beast'

It is important not to see the disease as a foreign invader, something beast-like to be loathed and despised. It is basically a bit of wrong programming in one or two of your body's systems, which unfortunately has the potential for serious consequences. Please don't hate your body for 'turning against' you. Human beings all have the capacity for disease. We were made with systems that are very easily sent out of kilter, and a small disturbance can have a devastating effect. In the end, who is afflicted by disease and who is not is largely a matter of chance. For the sake of your general well-being, you need to try hard to accept yourself in your new identity.

Emotional consequences of the diagnosis

In the early days of MS, a person will grieve for the loss of his or her health. This type of mourning is no different from the feelings of bereavement following the death of a person you were close to.

Grief is generally followed by denial, and then resistance. When these emotional states are accompanied by depression, it's no wonder you can feel bleak.

Grieving

You would not be human if you didn't grieve for your lost good health, your plans for the future and so on. However, grieving is healthy – it is the process that carries you through to eventual acceptance. Grieving also helps you to integrate your condition into your awareness of who you are as a person. The trouble is, you may at last have come to accept the presence of MS in your life when you are hit with another symptom or, worse still, a relapse that leaves you in a poorer physical state than before. Incorporating the new symptom into your new self may involve going through the grieving process again.

For the person with MS, it is natural to feel sad, angry and so on, because something of great importance has been stolen from you and been replaced with something else:

- You have lost the person you were, and instead have an identity that is bound up with disease.
- You have lost an active body and gained one that is being infiltrated with disease.
- You may lose effective functioning, at least temporarily, when you are used to being able to freely speak, write, cook, walk and so on.
- At times you may lose your energy and feel fatigue instead.
- You may lose control over what you do with your time, gaining a body that takes over that control.
- You are likely to lose much of your spontaneity, gaining the need to plan virtually every action.
- You may lose the full use of your limbs from time to time, gaining instead limbs that either refuse to work or have a will of their own.
- You have lost a natural relationship with other people, gaining a relationship with other people that is often loaded with sympathy, pity, anger, disappointment and so on.
- You are at risk of losing your self-confidence, to have it replaced by insecurity and vulnerability.

It's important to note, however, that grieving, and all the emotions bound up with grieving, is part of the process of adjusting to a chronic condition. To accelerate that adjustment period, follow these steps:

- Try to accept your grief as a healthy reaction to the losses you are expecting.
- Keeping your grief to yourself is not healthy and takes away from energy reserves that may already be depleted. Try to describe your innermost feelings to a few trusted people. It will make a difference.
- If you find opening up to others very difficult, ask for a referral to a counsellor or psychotherapist. Therapy can help you come to terms with your diagnosis.

Fear

Bound up with grief is generally fear, or at least great apprehension. However, it is normal to be afraid when you have a disease for which there is, as yet, no cure. Fears tend to centre around the future, and what will become of you. You are afraid of ending up in a wheelchair, of looking odd in society, of how far you might deteriorate, of losing all your friends, of becoming entirely dependent upon others, and even of the long-term effects of medication.

Chronic illness exerts profound effects on the individual. It is not always easy to be cheerful and bright when you have a cold, never mind a degenerative brain disease that manifests itself in odd and distressing ways. In most cases of MS, the fear of the unknown becomes far less pronounced with the passage of time as you learn that it is still possible to take pleasure from family life; that you can still enjoy social occasions; that you can still take up interests and hobbies; and that you can still be of use to others.

Denial

You may be surprised to learn that denial is part of the adaptive process. It is one of the normal emotions you pass through after the diagnosis, and, so long as it doesn't interfere with treatment and self-care, it can actually be a positive coping device. Some people are just not ready, emotionally, to face the truth, so cope by having 'time out'. You may not want to hear the words 'multiple sclerosis', neither may you want to discuss it or meet anyone else with the condition.

Resistance

In many, denial is followed by resistance. To prove to yourself that the disease won't impact greatly on your physical abilities, you may become very active, dashing here and there, taking up squash and going swimming twice a week. A part of you accepts that you have the disease, but the fighting part of you is determined to find a way to overcome it. This may also be done by zealously searching for information and advice, and poring over different treatments and suggested cures. To other people, your energy in this phase can be misinterpreted as anger. Indeed, when your doctor fails to have all the answers, you may find yourself shouting and be surprised at how angry you do, in fact, feel.

Adjustment

As time slowly passes, your resistance will normally die down and you should start to cope with the worst of your negative emotions, the feeling of being socially isolated and the uncertainty about the future. It is also a time when you are battling with yourself to let go of the past; when you are trying to convince yourself that you can find things in life to enjoy. Opening up to other people will help you to adjust.

Acceptance

In the final stage of the bereavement process, you should be able to accept that you and MS are inextricably linked, that it is a part of you and that life goes on. You are able now to think about other things, other people and really switch off. This has the effect of helping your family and friends to reach acceptance, too, because those close to you will have stumbled through the bereavement process every bit as much as you have.

The big problem with MS is that you can be sailing along, congratulating yourself on how well you're coping, when you're hit with a bad patch, a new symptom, or a relapse. You feel angry, frustrated, sad and anxious, but you have no choice but to come to terms with what is happening – maybe after experiencing all the stages of bereavement once more. For your emotional well-being, it is essential that you incorporate the bad patch, new symptom or relapse into your new identity, and once more get on with life. As time goes by, you'll become expert at adapting.

Getting stuck at one stage

Getting stuck at one stage of the bereavement process can result in people seeing themselves in a more negative light, which impinges on every aspect of their lives and the people in it. The only way out of this is to allow yourself to mourn for what you have lost. Allow yourself a good feeling-sorry-for-yourself cry, and with any luck the healing process will begin.

Living with MS is as much of a challenge to family and friends as it is to you. Indeed, in the early days they are almost certain to go through a similar gamut of emotions, beginning with grieving and ending at acceptance. When acceptance eludes them, however, they remain in a state of chronic frustration, anxiety and unhappiness, with an increased likelihood of being depressed. In this situation, it is best for everyone to openly discuss their concerns and any grievances. It is also important to listen to each other and respect each other's feelings and wishes. Talking and listening are always important when chronic disease becomes part of the picture. However, as well as sharing your concerns, it is important that you allow your family 'time out'.

Possible long-term emotions

Battling with negative emotions on occasion is, sadly, part and parcel of MS.

Feeling angry

Not only can anger be a central part of the bereavement process – usually related to resistance – it can rear its ugly head on occasions for many years to come. Anger and frustration are natural reactions to certain situations and can either be employed to hurt another person, or as a source of creative energy. It is likely to arise whenever the disease stops you doing something, when it makes you aware of being different, or when other people don't understand.

Partners of people with MS are also liable to experience anger – not only because they hate seeing you suffer, but also because their own plans for the future are now drastically changed.

When inability to perform an activity makes you angry and frustrated, try to avoid lashing out. It is not fair to make another person take the blame. If you can find healthy outlets for your anger, you will find yourself less anxious and stressed. Some people like to dig the garden, polish the car, or bake a batch of scones. If you are not able to burn off your anger in such a physical way, you can release the negative tension by giving one or two loud roars, banging your fist on the table, setting yourself to organizing a charity auction or singing a few jolly songs.

Feeling useless

MS can be a very limiting condition. Tasks once accomplished with ease now have to be carried out slowly and steadily, or dropped altogether – particularly during a relapse. Many jobs around the house have to be allocated to other family members – or to a paid cleaner. Onlookers may quip, 'Lucky you – having someone else do all that hard work!' They don't realize you would give anything to be able to clean the house thoroughly each and every day.

It is the same with many of the activities you previously enjoyed – and not necessarily ones requiring much effort. Many people with MS experience disabling fatigue, some suffer tremors or drag a leg, and these things can stop them from carrying out the most basic of functions. Sadly, some activities may now be permanently out of your scope, but others can be achieved given patience and time.

Also, it is important to your mental well-being that you make use of all the mobility aids and assistance devices available. Accept whatever practical support you need, then get on with maintaining and improving your quality of life. The sooner you accept help and support, the better your life can be.

Feeling vulnerable

Vulnerability is a natural human condition. We all need people to love us; we all crave the affirmation of others. To a large extent we are all dependent on others, measuring their responses in order to reassure ourselves that we are worthwhile human beings, that we are lovable. When people are chronically ill, they can feel unattractive and that they have little to offer the people around them. They can therefore feel they are no longer lovable.

Feelings of vulnerability will always be present in chronic illness, but you can defeat the worst of them by looking less to outsiders for affirmation. We all have inner strengths and particular talents, many of which we may be unaware of. Yet if we waited for others to point them out, we would likely be waiting for ever!

Your particular forte may be in planning and organizing, or problem solving, or handling finances within the family. You may be an authority on steam engines, an inspired cook, a good listener, a talented artist, an excellent singer, a diligent student, a competent driver, etc. etc. Please do not underestimate yourself!

Feeling guilty

It is natural to want to blame your state of health on someone. However, many people place the blame at their own doors, imagining they must have done something very wrong to deserve what they see as retribution. But blaming either yourself or others is pointless, and you don't want to add to your burdens in this way.

Guilt also arises when you feel you are a burden on members of your family. You feel bad about their extra workload, and because their free time is now more limited. When people with MS need 'full-time' carers, it is important that the carers have time to themselves, that they retain some interests, and take occasional 'time off'. The knowledge that they are enjoying their lives regardless of your ill health and limitations – which, of course, they have a perfect right to do – should help you to feel less guilty.

Overcoming stress

Low self-esteem, persistent tiredness and anxiety about the future – not to mention disturbing symptoms and the onset of a relapse – can cause a build-up of emotional stress. However, there are ways to help you shake off the stress and develop a more positive outlook.

Living in the present

A calm and contented *now* is more emotionally nourishing than a mind reeling with the upsets the future may hold. In the same way, cherishing the moment is preferable to letting it slip by unappreciated because you are too busy thinking ahead. How many of us look forward to seeing a film, a band, a show, a play – but don't think to enjoy the journey there? How many of us look forward to summer, forgetting to appreciate spring?

But, you may ask, is it possible for someone with MS to master the art of living in the present? What is the alternative – to sit brooding on how things used to be, how they might now be, if only . . . ? Wouldn't it be better to read a gripping book, pen a poem, surf the internet, take a walk, or have a cuddle with that special someone?

Finding new challenges

As well as offering distraction, taking on a new challenge can be infinitely rewarding. It can also help you to feel more positive about yourself. Consider taking up oil-painting, stencilling, playing the keyboard, tapestry-work, glass and china painting, picture-framing, jewellery-making – the list is endless.

Learning something different can prove very satisfying too. Maybe you might like to acquire a few academic qualifications, or enrol in a leisure interest course (where the atmosphere is more informal and regular attendance not so important). Studying a subject that is helpful in dealing with MS – for example, homeopathy, yoga, reflexology, aromatherapy, meditation, relaxation, stress management, assertiveness training, etc. – may prove invaluable. It would also give you the opportunity to help other people.

However, it is important that you choose an activity or study course that really interests you, and that you expect to do well at. Failure can be difficult to handle when you are also attempting to come to terms with the condition. Don't forget to congratulate yourself on each small success along the way.

Chronic stress

Chronic stress is the state of being constantly 'on alert'. The physiological changes associated with this state – that is, a fast heart-rate, shallow breathing, and muscle tension – persist over a long period, making relaxation very difficult. Chronic stress can lead to nerviness, hypertension, irritability and depression.

The condition commonly arises when any of the following needs fail to be met on a long-term basis:

The need to be understood

People with MS need to feel that the people close to them understand their concerns about the future. When you suspect people think you are worrying unnecessarily, you can feel so upset and isolated you begin to shut others out. Unfortunately, it is not always easy for others to understand how you feel. Take a deep breath and calmly share your feelings. However, if you have repeatedly tried to help certain people understand and they are still upsetting you, tell them calmly how they are making you feel. Hopefully, this will shock them into seeing the situation from your point of view. If not, it would probably be more beneficial to your state of mind to cut yourself off from these people, if possible.

The need to be loved

Feeling unlovable is one of the greatest threats to the emotional well-being of people with MS. You may worry that the emotional and physical burdens will be too heavy for your partner and he or she may ultimately end the relationship – and that may cause you subconsciously to withdraw your affections. You may even wonder how anyone *could* love a person with a degenerative disease, who walks oddly and is always tired. The fear of being unlovable may even have made you irrational and antagonistic.

Before you can be loved by others, you need to love yourself. You need to see yourself as a worthwhile person with qualities that you, as well as others, can respect. Don't let apathy rule. Start the way you mean to go on by taking the following action:

- Make a list of your ten best physical attributes.
- Make a list of your ten best character traits.
- If physically possible, do at least one nice thing (however small) for another person each day. Don't forget to congratulate yourself for it.
- Make the very most of your appearance, every minute of the day.
- Regularly treat yourself to a therapy you find uplifting (a reflexology massage, for example).
- Try to frequently indulge in something that stimulates your mind as well as creating a sense of fulfilment.

The need to love

MS can cause you to wholly focus on your symptoms, ultimately making you withdraw from the people around you. However, loving others and actively attempting to lighten their mood can have a positive impact on your own state of mind. For example, encouraging your partner to smile will make you smile too, phoning a friend with relationship problems can make you feel good about yourself, and showing interest in your lonely neighbour's vegetable patch can hearten you both. It doesn't need to take much either. You can make someone smile with a few carefully chosen words, and a bit of honest flattery will make you feel just as good as the recipient. He or she will likely be pleased and uplifted by the effort you have made, and hopefully will want to respond in kind. You have to give before you can hope to receive.

The need to be yourself

The roles many of us play out, perhaps unawares, often have their origins in early childhood. If, for example, the parents of a young woman – we'll call her Sophie – were always scathing about incompetence, she would probably grow up with the same mental attitude, going so far as to hide instances when she was less than perfect. Only when Sophie moves in with a partner who is far from perfect, a partner who is maybe even intimidated by her apparent 'perfection', will she begin to see that it is all right to be flawed.

There may be several ways in which you hide your real self. You may, for example, have dated a person who lived and breathed football. You liked them a lot, so skimmed through some of the sports pages and feigned an interest. But, realistically, going through life pretending to be interested in something you don't care a jot about causes untold inner stress. It is far better to be yourself, warts and all. This not only minimizes stress, it ensures that you know that the people important to you like you for who you really are.

The need to feel well

Constantly being anxious and despondent can make a person with MS feel unwell. Fatigue, face pain, leg numbness and mood swings (forgive me if these are not your particular symptoms) will only add to that feeling. However, taking positive steps to tackle the disease should counter the feeling of unwellness. For instance, you can improve matters by starting to eat healthily; taking regular exercise of some kind; avoiding exposure to harmful toxins; forging satisfactory relationships with your doctor, family and friends; learning the art of positive thinking; trying different complementary therapies; and taking a course in, for example, scenic photography. The feeling that you are actively helping yourself creates a sense of achievement and lowers stress levels.

Stress management

Stress can exacerbate the symptoms of MS, cause relapses, and accelerate the course of the disease. It arises not only as a result of what happens to a person, but also from their reactions to what happens. Negative inbred attitudes can actually cause people to see catastrophe in what to others would be normal, everyday events. When a situation is interpreted as a crisis, adrenaline is released into the bloodstream and the body automatically puts itself 'on alert'. Breathing becomes shallow and fast, the heart-rate quickens, blood pressure rises, and the muscles tense – allowing the person to deal with an emergency far more effectively. However, this response can be destructive when it occurs frequently, over a prolonged period of time.

In one study, a group of MS patients provided emotional support to other MS patients as part of a telephone intervention programme. The people giving support showed significant improvements in their confidence, self-awareness, self-esteem and depression. The people receiving support also showed improvements, but not quite as great as in the other group. This suggests that a sense of control and connection is very important in MS.

Delay your reaction

Because living with a chronic condition naturally creates stress in daily life, people with MS experience higher levels of stress than those without MS. However, you should find that curbing your responses to events can reduce the build-up of stress. As a troublesome event unfolds, try not to instantly react. Allow yourself the time to evaluate the situation; to see it as it really is. Now select a response that doesn't create more stress.

Life stress evaluation

If you take the time to evaluate all the relationships and activities in your everyday life, you will likely find some that induce a good deal more stress than benefit. Remember, however, that personal interactions will always produce a certain amount of stress. It is when the stress outweighs the positive gains that you need to consider limiting or ceasing that involvement.

Helping others to understand

In attempting to help the people you care about to understand the challenges you face with MS, you should try to be as honest and open as possible. You will find it far from easy to speak openly of your worries for the future, so think first about what you want to say. The following pointers should help you.

Communicating effectively

Before trying to describe your feelings about MS, you first need to focus on how you actually feel. Admitting to feeling guilty, frustrated, angry, resentful, useless, etc. will be hard, even to yourself, but doing so will help you to come to terms with those feelings, and ultimately to let them go. Sharing your feelings with others, meanwhile, is an important step towards halting the problems that those feelings can cause.

Try to be wary of making assumptions about how other people feel about you – for example, 'I know you think I'm worrying too much and that makes me really upset', or 'I don't believe you could really love someone who might end up in a wheelchair, and that makes me feel sad', or 'All you can say is "life's hard", and that makes me feel as if you don't understand one bit'. Such comments will be seen as unfair judgements, or accusations; they may even provoke a quarrel.

Speaking directly of your 'emotional problems' – without implying that the other person is contributing to those problems – will help that person to take your comments more seriously. It should encourage him or her to be more thoughtful and caring. However, there may be times when conflict arises, when someone upsets you by doing or saying something insensitive. In such instances, consider the following before you reply:

- Ensure you have interpreted the other person's behaviour correctly. For example, you may view your mother bringing you a basket of fruit and vegetables as a criticism of your diet – when in truth it is to show that she cares. You have a perfect right to interpret the words or actions of others in whatever way you wish, but that interpretation is not necessarily reality. In fact, it is amazing how wrong we often are in our perceptions of what others think and feel.
- Make sure you are specific in recalling another person's behaviour. For example, 'You never understand when I tell you how physically tired I feel' is far more inflammatory than 'You didn't seem to understand yesterday when I said I felt physically tired'.
- Be sure that what you are about to say is what you really mean. For example, statements such as 'Everyone thinks you're insensitive' or 'We all think you've got an attitude problem' are, besides being inflammatory, incredibly unfair. We have no way of knowing that 'everyone' is of the same opinion. The use of the depersonalized 'everyone', 'we' or 'us' – often said in the hope of deflecting the listener's anger – can cause far more hurt and anger than if the criticism is direct and personal.

It is easy to see how others can misunderstand or take offence when we fail to communicate effectively. Changing the habits of a lifetime is far from easy, however. It means analysing our thoughts before rearranging them into speech. We are rewarded for our efforts, though, when those close to us start to *really* listen, when they cease to be annoyed as we carefully explain something they had not fully understood.

Dealing with unfair comments

Sarcastic and derisory remarks from others can chip away at your confidence. They should not, therefore, pass unchallenged. Standing up for yourself is not always easy, but doing so can have a releasing effect – unlike when you fake indifference, or clam up and walk away. In such instances, you may end up feeling hurt, offended and very resentful. Your most intense feeling, however, will likely be that of anger – at the other person, and at yourself, for allowing yourself to be hurt.

For example, if your partner were to say, 'You never want to watch sci-fi films with me these days. I wish you were more like you used to be', you could calmly answer, 'That's quite hurtful, you know. I still love sci-fi, but can't watch it because the flashing lights hurt my eyes. I'm the same person I always was, but with a few limitations.'

Or, when someone you don't know too well comments on your walking, you could answer calmly, 'If I didn't have to drag my leg, I wouldn't – believe me.' In response, the person may well be sympathetic, giving you the opportunity to reveal more of your symptoms if you wish. If the person is probing in a way you find distasteful, you would be best advised to say something like, 'I don't actually want to discuss this right now.' Adding an excuse such as 'I'm in a hurry' may soften the punch, while allowing you to keep your dignity.

Your relationships

People with MS need to know that the people close to them care. Most of all they crave the understanding of their nearest and dearest, feeling upset when they are shown impatience or lack of thought.

Partnerships

Naturally, most partners want the very best for their loved one. A small percentage of partners may decide it is all too much for them to handle and end the relationship – though this type of person would likely prove unsupportive and the relationship falter at some point anyway. We are all different in how we react to and handle problems. Some people are unable to cope with illness; others may have been looking for an excuse to leave, and find this excuse in MS. Statistics show that only a small majority of partners leave, however.

Take time to calmly talk problems through. Exchanging percep-tions, fears and needs carries the bonus of strengthening your relationship. If your relationship is on a downhill spiral and you are finding it impossible to open up to one another, counselling is probably your best option. Here are some suggestions:

- Make a pact that you will try hard to work together to come to terms with MS. The relationship may falter if either partner fails to accept its existence.
- Work on how you speak to one another, opening channels of communication as much as possible. Once you are freely able to

discuss such things as feelings, bodily functions and sexual matters, your problems will be so much easier to deal with. If you find it difficult to communicate effectively with one another, try reading books on communication, take a course on communication skills, or see a trained counsellor.

- Have the courage to be yourself. Remember that you have the right to be the person you are, and to be different from other people. You also have the right to feel what you feel and to ask for your needs to be met. Hiding your feelings and needs because you fear what people might think of you can not only stifle your personality, it can raise your stress levels too.

- Acknowledge that your partner has feelings and needs. He or she has a perfect right to be tired of pushing the wheelchair or of your complaints about your vision, and has a right to tell you so. When you start to be honest with one another and respect one another's needs, your relationship will become stronger.

The caregiver

Many people with MS need long-term physical, financial and psychological support from partner, family and friends. Very often, one person is the prime caregiver – therefore, the good mental and physical health of that person is vital. When the burden is considerable, the mental and physical health of both patient and caregiver can be threatened. Indeed, it is said that the more hours dedicated to the patient, the more depressed is the caregiver. As a result, the care of the caregiver is diminished, which impacts on his or her ability to function.

In one study, caregivers said the most distressing aspect of MS was the psychological impact of the condition on the patient and the incurability of the disease. In their opinion, the best form of support was practical help, in the shape of cooking, cleaning and so on. Better availability of medical and financial advice came a close second.

Support groups

There are now numerous local MS support groups, offering meetings, information, and the ability to borrow or buy available books and audio-visual resources from the group library. Many support groups book guest speakers, such as physiotherapists, benefits specialists, occupational therapists, complementary therapies experts, etc. More importantly, the meetings present a wonderful opportunity for fellow sufferers to get together and have a good chat. Mutual support is greatly beneficial, and life-long friends can be made.

References

Bansil, S. *et al.*, 'Multiple sclerosis: pathogenesis and treatment', *Seminars in Neurology*, June 1994, 14(2): 146–53.

Belluzzi, A. *et al.*, 'Effect of an enteric-coated fish oil preparation on relapses in Crohn's disease', *New England Journal of Medicine*, 1996, 334: 1557–616.

Bray, P. F. *et al.*, 'Antibodies against Epstein-Barr nuclear antigen (EBNA) in multiple sclerosis CSF, and two pentapeptide sequence identities between EBNA and myelin basic protein', *Neurology*, September 1992, 42: 1798–804.

Erasmus, Udo, *Fats that Heal, Fats that Kill*. Alive Books, Burnaby, British Columbia, 1993.

Fazekas, F. *et al.*, 'Randomised placebo-controlled trial of monthly intravenous immunoglobulin therapy in relapsing-remitting multiple sclerosis', *Lancet*, 1997, 349: 589–93.

Francis, D. A. *et al.*, 'Multiple sclerosis in north-east Scotland', *Brain*, 1987, 110: 181–96.

Frohman, E. *et al.*, 'Disease modifying agent-related skin reactions in multiple sclerosis: prevention, assessment and management', *Multiple Sclerosis*, 2004, 10: 302–7.

Herndon, R. M. *et al.*, 'Pathology and pathophysiology of multiple sclerosis', *Seminars in Neurology*, 1985, 5: 99–106.

Joyce, M. *et al.*, 'Reflexology helps multiple sclerosis', *Journal of Alternative and Complementary Medicine*, July 1997: 10–12.

Kleijjnen, J. *et al.*, *Lancet*, 1992, 340: 8828.

Kupparanjan, K. *et al.*, 'Effect of Ashwagandha on the process of ageing in human volunteers', *Journal of Research in Ayurveda and Sadai*, 1980: 247–58.

Larner, A. J. *et al.*, 'Aetiological role of viruses in multiple sclerosis: a review', *Journal of the Royal Society of Medicine*, 1986, 79: 412–17.

Miller, D. *et al.*, 'A controlled trial of natalizumab for relapsing-remitting multiple sclerosis', *New England Journal of Medicine*, 2003, 348: 15–23.

Poser, C. M. *et al.*, 'New diagnostic criteria for multiple sclerosis:

guidelines for research protocols', *Annals of Neurology*, 1983, 13: 227–30.

Poser, C. M., 'Pathogenesis of multiple sclerosis', *Acta Neuropathology*, 1986, 71: 1–10.

Rorke, W. W., 'Results of homeopathic treatment in a well-defined and well-known chronic nervous disease', *British Homeopathy Journal*, 1925, 25: 131–44.

Sibley, W. A., 'Management of the patient with multiple sclerosis', *Annals of Neurology*, 1985, 5: 134–45.

Siev-Ner, I. *et al.*, 'Reflexology significantly improves parasthesia, urinary symptoms and spasticity in people with multiple sclerosis', *Multiple Sclerosis*, 2003, 9: 356–61.

Warot, D. *et al.*, 'Comparative effects of ginkgo biloba extracts on psychomotor performance in healthy subjects', *Therapie*, 1991, 46 (1): 33–6.

Weiner, H., 'When nerves break down', *New Scientist*, 2004, 182, 2450: 44–7.

Zajicek, J. *et al.*, *Lancet*, 2003, 263: 1517–26.

Useful addresses

United Kingdom

The Multiple Sclerosis Resource Centre
7 Peartree Business Centre
Peartree Road
Stanway
Colchester
Essex CO3 0JN
Tel.: 0800 783 0518 (then press 1)
Fax: 01206 505449
Website: www.msrc.co.uk

This charitable organization offers a web advice resource and 24-hour telephone support service. The website has a message board, chat room and bi-monthly magazine. The telephone service offers counselling and support. The website is also the home of the Best Bet Diet Group, giving recipes, testimonials and information about supplements.

Multiple Sclerosis (MS) Society
MS National Centre
372 Edgware Road
Cricklewood
London NW2 6ND
Tel.: 020 8438 0700
Fax: 020 8438 0701
Helpline: 0808 800 8000 (9 a.m. to 9 p.m., Monday to Friday)
Information helpline: 020 8438 0799 (10 a.m. to 3 p.m., Monday to Friday)
Website: www.mssociety.org.uk
Email: info@mssociety.org.uk

The MS Society is the largest UK charitable organization for people with MS, with around 85,000 members and a network of over 350 local UK branches. The MS National Centre provides information and support to anyone affected by MS. It is a source of authoritative advice, a place where learning and teaching about MS can be shared, and a focal point for the UK-wide MS Society. All calls to the MS Society national helpline are free and completely confidential. The society's specialist staff and trained volunteers are available to support you whatever your concern. There are offices in Northern Ireland and Scotland as well: see below.

Action MS (Northern Ireland)
Belfast Office
Knockbracken Healthcare Park
Saintfield Road
Belfast BT8 8BH
Northern Ireland
Tel.: 028 907 907 07
Fax: 028 9040 2010
Helpline: 0800 028 88 33
Website: www.actionms.co.uk
Email: info@actionms.co.uk

This action group offers all the latest information about MS. There is a free helpline, fundraising events, a regular newsletter and several affiliated regional support groups.

Multiple Sclerosis Society
Scotland Office
Ratho Park
88 Glasgow Road
Ratho Station
Newbridge EH28 8PP
Tel.: 0131 335 4050
Fax: 0131 335 4051

www.msdecisions.org.uk

This website offers a great deal of information on every aspect of MS.

Bioflow Magnotherapy
P.O. Box 135
Copt Hall Road
Lightham
Sevenoaks
Kent TN15 9WZ
Tel.: 0870 766 9739
Website: www.ecomagnets.com
Email: sales@ecomagnets.com

British Homeopathic Association
Hahnemann House
29 Park Street West
Luton LU1 3BE
Tel.: 0870 444 3950
Fax: 0870 444 3960
Website: www.trusthomeopathy.org

British Herbal Medicine Association
The Secretary
1 Wickham Road
Boscombe
Bournemouth
Dorset BH7 6JX
Tel.: 01202 433691
Fax: 01202 417079
Website: www.bhma.info
Email: secretary@bhma.info

British Reflexology Association
Administration Office
Monks Orchard
Whitbourne
Worcester WR6 5RB
Tel.: 01886 821207
Fax: 01886 822017
Website: www.britreflex.co.uk
Email: bra@britreflex.co.uk

124

Motability Operations
City Gate House
22 Southwark Bridge Road
London SE1 9HB
Tel.: 0845 456 4566
Website: www.motability.co.uk

For Motability car scheme.

Register of Chinese Herbal Medicine
Office 5
Ferndale Business Centre
1 Exeter Street
Norwich NR2 4QB
Tel.: 01603 667557
Website: www.rchm.co.uk
Email: herbmed@rchm.co.uk

The best time to telephone is 9 a.m. to 5 p.m., Monday to Friday (answerphone at other times).

The Register of Chinese Herbal Medicine (RCHM) is a UK professional body that represents over 400 fully qualified practitioners of Chinese herbal medicine. For details of your nearest member, please contact the above address.

route2mobility
Newbury Road
Enham Alamein
Andover
Hants. SP11 6JS
Tel.: 0845 60 762 60
Website: www.motability.co.uk

For Motability wheelchairs and scooters scheme.

USEFUL ADDRESSES

Overseas

National Multiple Sclerosis Society
733 Third Avenue
New York
NY 10017-5706
Tel.: 212 986 3240 or 800 FIGHT MS or 800 344 4867
Website: www.nationalmssociety.org

This is the primary resource for MS in the USA. It has periodic compilations of current research, pamphlets covering symptoms and other MS issues, and a library with medical journals used to provide information to patients and professionals. The society publishes *Inside MS* magazine. Its website is excellent.

Multiple Sclerosis Association of America
706 Haddonfield Road
Cherry Hill
NJ 08002
Tel.: 856 488 4500 or 800 532 7667
Website: www.msaa.com
This organization offers direct patient care services, including equipment loans. It makes referrals, publishes reports, and offers a newsletter.

Multiple Sclerosis Foundation, Inc.
6350 North Andrews Avenue
Fort Lauderdale
FL 33309-2130
Tel.: 954 776 6805 or 800 225 6495
Website: www.msfacts.org

This group provides information on both alternative and traditional treatments for MS. Patients should investigate any non-traditional therapies thoroughly and discuss them with their doctor.

Multiple Sclerosis Society of Canada
175 Bloor Street
East Suite 700
North Tower
Toronto
Ontario M4W 3R8
Tel.: 416 922 6065
Fax: 416 922 7538
Website: www.mssociety.ca
Email: info@mssociety.ca

This society gives MS information, advice and the latest research results. It aims to provide hope for the future through support of MS research into the cause, treatment and cure of the disease, and hope for today through its many services that assist people with MS and their families. The website provides links to local groups throughout Canada.

Herb Research Foundation (HRF)
4140 15th Street
Boulder
CO 80304
Tel.: 303 449 2265 or voice mail 800 748 2617
Website: www.herbs.org

HRF provides scientific information about the health effects of herbs. Reports, research abstracts, a phone hotline and other services are available for a fee.

Index